STOP

BREA

BE

IT

D0379879

OTHER BOOKS BY DR. SAMUEL EPSTEIN

The Mutagenicity of Pesticides (M.I.T. Press, 1971)

Drugs of Abuse: Their Genetic and Other Chronic Nonpsychiatric Hazards (M.I.T. Press, 1971)

The Legislation of Product Safety (M.I.T. Press, 1974)

The Politics of Cancer (Sierra Club Books, 1978)

Hazardous Wastes in America (Sierra Club Books, 1982)

Cancer in Britain: The Politics of Prevention (Pluto Press, 1983)

The Safe Shopper's Bible (MacMillan Publishing Company, 1995)

The Breast Cancer Prevention Program (MacMillan Publishing Company, 1997; Second Edition, 1998)

The Politics of Cancer, Revisited (East Ridge Press, 1998)

GOT Genetically Engineered MILK! The Monsanto rBGH/BST Milk Wars Handbook (Seven Stories Press, 2001)

Unreasonable Risk: How to Avoid Cancer from Cosmetics and Personal Care Products: The Neways Story (Environmental Toxicology, 2001)

The Stop Cancer Before It Starts Campaign: How to Win the Losing War Against Cancer (2003)

Unreasonable Risk: How to Avoid Cancer from Cosmetics and Personal Care Products: The Neways Story (Environmental Toxicology, 2005)

Cancer-Gate: How to Win the Losing Cancer War (Baywood Publishing Company, Inc., 2005)

Shopper Beware: How to Avoid Cancer and Other Toxic Effects from Cosmetics and Personal Care Products (Japan: Lyon-sha Publishing, 2006)

What's In Your Milk? (Trafford Publishing, 2006)

Healthy Beauty (BenBella Books, 2010)

National Cancer Institute and American Cancer Society: Criminal Indifference to Cancer Prevention and Conflicts of Interest (Xlibris Publishing, 2011)

Good Clean Food (Skyhorse Publishing, 2013)

STOP
BREAST CANCER
BEFORE
IT STARTS

Samuel S. Epstein, MD

Research Assistant
Alessandra Gibson, MPH, MBA

Seven Stories Press
New York

Seven Stories Press
140 Watts Street
New York, NY 10013
www.sevenstories.com

College professors may order examination copies of Seven Stories Press titles for a free. To order, visit http://www.sevenstories.com/textbook or send a fax on school letterhead to (212) 226-1411.

Book design by Jon Gilbert

Library of Congress Cataloging-in-Publication Data

Epstein, Samuel S.
  Stop breast cancer before it starts / Samuel S. Epstein, M.D.—A Seven Stories Press first edition.
    pages cm
  ISBN 978-1-60980-488-6 (pbk.)
  1. Breast--Cancer. 2. Breast--Cancer--Prevention. 3. Women--Health and hygiene. 4. Health promotion--Evaluation. I. Title.
  RC280.B8E665 2013
  616.99'449--dc23
                                2013017531
Printed in the United States

9 8 7 6 5 4 3 2 1

To my wondrous wife, Catherine,
who makes all things possible.

Contents

Abbreviations **ix**

Foreword by Joseph Mercola, D.O., F.A.C.N. **xi**

Introduction by Rosalie Bertell, PhD **1**

Chapter 1: The Escalating Incidence of Breast Cancer **5**

Chapter 2: Avoidable Causes of Breast Cancer **25**

Chapter 3: Mammography **41**

Chapter 4: Newspaper Articles, 1992–2002 **57**

Chapter 5: Press Releases & Huffington Post Blog Posts, 1992–2011 **79**

Appendix A: The American Cancer Society's Reckless, If Not Criminal, Track Record on Prevention of Breast and Other Cancers **193**

Appendix B: Breast Carcinogens Listed in the 2010 American Cancer Society (ACS) Report as "Needing More Study" **199**

Appendix C: National Academy of Sciences December 2011 Report on Avoidable Causes of Breast Cancer **201**

Appendix D: Citizen Petitions to the Food and Drug Administration Authored by Dr. Epstein **203**

Acknowledgments **219**

About the Author **221**

Abbreviations

ACS	American Cancer Society
BSE	breast self-examination
CBE	clinical breast examination
CPSC	Consumer Product Safety Commission
DCIS	Ductal Carcinoma In Situ
EPA	Environmental Protection Agency
ERT	estrogen replacement therapy
FDA	Food and Drug Administration
FY	Fiscal Year
GE	Genetically Engineered
HGH	Human Growth Hormone
IARC	International Agency for Research on Cancer
ICI	Imperial Chemical Industry
IGF-1	Insulin-like Growth Factor 1
NAS	National Academy of Sciences
NBCAM	National Breast Cancer Awareness Month
NDA	New Drug Application
NCI	National Cancer Institute
OC	Oral Contraceptives
OSHA	Occupational Safety Health Administration
RAD	Radiation Absorbed Dose
rBGH	Recombinant Bovine Growth Hormone
USPSTF	United States Preventive Services Task Force

Foreword

If you are a woman, there is a one in eight chance you will develop invasive breast cancer in your lifetime, as breast cancer is the most common cancer in women with nearly a quarter million new cases diagnosed in 2011. Interestingly, 99 percent of breast cancer patients have chemicals called parabens in their breast cancer tissue.

Parabens are problematic as they have estrogen-like properties that are widely known to promote the development of breast cancer. Any time you shampoo your hair or apply deodorant, body lotion, or cosmetics, there's a good chance you're also absorbing your fair share of the estrogen-mimicking, cancer-promoting compounds they likely contain.

Sadly, this is only one of the environmental exposures that may increase your risk of developing breast cancer.

There are many others, from hair dyes and hormonal contraceptives, to synthetic hormones in milk and even the very procedure *recommended* for breast cancer screening—mammography. Certainly there are breast cancer cases that occur as the result of genetics or manifest even in the absence of a known environmental or other trigger, but for the most part these numbers are dwarfed by the influences for which we have enormous control over.

There is strong support that some of these epigenetic regulators could be the carcinogens in your food, water, air, and workplace. They're all around you, yet the warnings—and the regulatory actions—have been slim to nonexistent.

As the chairman of the Cancer Prevention Coalition, and professor emeritus of Environmental and Occupational Medicine at the University of Illinois at Chicago School of Public Health, there is perhaps no better authority to speak on this urgent issue than Samuel Epstein, MD. Why are we losing the war against cancer when it is very clearly a "winnable" one? This is the question Dr. Epstein answers in this book that should be on every woman's nightstand. As he points out: "Being able to cure a disease should be secondary to preventing it in the first place . . ."

THE WAR AGAINST CANCER *CAN* BE WON

Having authored 270 scientific articles and twenty books on the causes and prevention of cancer, Dr. Epstein is exceptionally qualified to discuss topics related to cancer prevention, and the toxicological causes of cancer that *must* be part of any effective cancer prevention plan.

We have been engaged in the "war against cancer" for more than forty years and have not made any progress in preventing deaths from breast cancer. If you carefully examine the practice of the cancer industry, it becomes very obvious that it is a well-oiled machine that is more focused on generating large profits than long-term cures.

Even the American Cancer Society, the US organization perhaps most associated with the war against cancer, has received funding from manufacturers of cancer-causing products, and has in its history *opposed* regulations for products, like hair dyes, that contain cancer-causing ingredients. They are a part of the problem, not the solution. The Susan G. Komen Foundation is another glaring example of the massive conflict of interest in this area.

Beyond this, the facts about the cancer-causing chemicals and technologies being used widely in the United States—like nanoparticles in cosmetics that are becoming known as "universal asbestos"—are being hidden and ignored. You and your family use these products unaware of the risks they pose because you have been kept in the dark about their true toxic effects. Simple warnings on product labels could make all the difference, but for now you have to fend for yourself.

IF YOU'VE EVER TAKEN HORMONAL BIRTH CONTROL OR HAD A MAMMOGRAM . . .

You may remember, back in 2002, one of the largest and best-designed federal studies of hormone replacement therapy was halted because it was found that women taking these synthetic hormones had a greater risk of breast cancer, heart attack, stroke, and blood clots. The study made headlines because millions of women were *already* taking these synthetic hormones, and fortunately, it prompted many of them to quit.

WHAT DOES THIS HAVE TO DO WITH THE PILL?

Birth control pills contain the *same* types of synthetic hormones—estrogen and progestin—that were used in the cautionary study. What is needed is a similar wake-up call to the one that occurred in 2002, a warning that will prompt women to quit taking the pill, and this is what Dr. Epstein has provided in this book. It's *the* canary in the coalmine, showing, in black and white, facts that many of the products you most likely assumed to be safe are anything but.

Of particular importance are the sections on mammography screening—"a profit-driven technology posing risks compounded by unreliability," as Dr. Epstein so eloquently puts it.

Besides the fact that the ionizing radiation delivered during mammography can cause cancer in and of itself, overdiagnosis of cancer as well as misdiagnosis have been shown to be significant problems plaguing this form of cancer screening. And you are likely not aware that mammograms are especially inaccurate for women with dense breasts, and because of that, other screening tools are recommended. Certain states have already passed laws requiring women with dense breasts to be informed they may need to seek alternative screening methods—another glaring example that what you don't know can indeed hurt you.

What Dr. Epstein is offering in *Stop Breast Cancer Before it Starts* is an outstanding resource to educate you about the causes of this problem and, more importantly, provide you with the tools and information to make simple choices that can profoundly and radically decrease your risk of experiencing or dying from this disease, which currently afflicts nearly one in eight women.

—Joseph Mercola, D.O., F.A.C.N.
Founder of Mercola.com, the world's
most visited natural health website, and
New York Times best-selling author

Introduction

There are many factors in daily life that are directly associated with the development of breast cancer. Clearly it is critical that women be told about them and be encouraged to avoid them. Anyone who has followed this concern since the 1970s, when the increase in the rate of breast cancer and its earlier occurrence in some women became alarming to the public, knows it to be contentious.

The earliest medical attempt to address the problem involved very early models of mammography (X-ray machines designed specifically for imaging the breast), poor reading of nuclear radiation literature, and a public disagreement between scientists and health professionals over the merits of this new technology. We now know that the researchers had misinterpreted the dose-response data from the nuclear industry, and the original plan would likely have caused twelve breast cancers for every breast cancer it picked up early. This program was scrapped but only after quite a bit of damage was done to public relations. When it was reintroduced with reduced exposures, it has continued to be plagued with disagreements: Should insurance cover it? Is early diagnosis beneficial? Does it overdiagnose causing unnecessary distress and medical procedures? Is it OK to cause one breast cancer in order to detect another earlier? Many ethicists are uncomfortable with a medical test designed to prevent breast cancer death while causing breast cancer in some women who otherwise would not have had it. Some feminists worry that women's health care could be ignored by men's allocation of priority money spending on other medical needs if women do not fight for it. Some scientists question, on scientific grounds, whether there is really a benefit of any kind with this technology. Obviously dialogue across these issues has been difficult!

The reality is that the mammography program is a very lucrative business that is now well established, ready to fight any attempt to curb it.

Women who are wary of the high costs are now demanding that mammography be funded by health insurance plans. Most do not understand the periodic newspaper articles recommending that it not be used to screen premenopausal women or that screening be reduced to every two or three years rather than every year. They look to the American Cancer Society (ACS) and the National Cancer Institute (NCI) for guidance.

Dr. Samuel Epstein has been a pioneer in pointing out the lobbying and inside profiteering on the part of these two generally trusted agencies. The NCI and the ACS are lobbied by the drug and medical instrument manufacturers, funded by the industries and professional agencies, and have been governed for many years by radiologists. Women are unaware that these agencies have been censured by Congressional committees for biased advertising, giving misleading advice to women, and non-factual promotion of technology.

Unfortunately, cancer has become a billion-dollar business, and its primary compassionate goal of healing, let alone prevention, is taking a back seat to survival as an industry.

I hope that the reader will keep an open mind and even seek more information if needed in order to reach a reasonable conclusion. What I have outlined for mammography also relates to the chemical, food, and nuclear industries. You will also find many household items that are hazardous to your health written up in this book, as well as detrimental pharmaceuticals and beauty products against which you have seen no warnings! Being able to cure a disease should be secondary to preventing it in the first place—even though there is little glory (or money) in the latter. You can use this book as a resource guide to purchases and a check list for your bathroom medicine cabinet.

Since we are no longer able to blame germs for all human illness, the causes of cancer need to be found either in one's genetic endowment or environment. Without microbes to blame, we are left with real people creating hazardous products or spewing toxic waste into the air, streams, or landfills. Naming the perpetrator will bring cries of "innocence" with multimillion-dollar campaigns to "prove" it!

There is good information available—but it does not come with bells and whistles and bundles of funding. It takes conscientious reading and study to ferret out the truth—but is it always worth this effort? Please read on, cross check information (not propaganda), and adopt the sensible ways to avoid environmental factors known to influence breast cancer. Campaigns for breast examination clinics and particularly for lessons in self-examination rather than relying on mammography would be more reasonable. You know more about your breasts than a mammography machine does! It is time to take charge of your own life and health! Remember that the consumer has the power to affect the producer, shape the market around true needs, and note products that are harmful. It is the time for women to exercise this powerful responsibly!

Consumer products are a part of the human-constructed environment which women are able to avoid if they are prewarned. Other parts of the environment are not as easily avoided and might involve deeper life changes or more political involvement. However, the first important step toward self-protection is to gain knowledge about the dangers. Dr. Epstein has provided this guide to make the first step easy!

On behalf of the many health professionals who personally choose not to belong to a mammography screening program, and who avoid, where possible, the other environmental hazards known to be associated with breast cancer, I would like to thank Dr. Epstein for his perseverance with factual advice over some thirty decades of struggle! I am glad that his remarkable career has now been properly recognized by the United Nations Program to halt the further spread of cancers globally!

—The late Rosalie Bertell, PhD
Former President of the International
Institute of Concern for Public Health, Toronto, Canada
Regent of the International Physicians for
Humanitarian Medicine, Geneva, Switzerland

CHAPTER 1

The Escalating Incidence of Breast Cancer

According to the National Academy of Sciences, breast cancer has long been the most common invasive cancer among women in the USA,[1] accounting for an estimated 229,000 new cases in 2012.[2] It is the most commonly diagnosed cancer in women under fifty. As of January 2002, nearly 2.3 million women were living with the disease. On average, girls born today have about a 12 percent risk of developing breast cancer in their lifetime.[3] After lung cancer, it is the second most common cause of women's cancer mortality,[4] with about 40,030 deaths expected in 2013.[5]

ESTIMATED NEW BREAST CANCER CASES AND DEATHS

Year	New cases	Deaths
2009	194,280	40,610
2010	209,060	40,230
2011	232,620	39,970
2012	229,060	39,920
2013	234,580	40,030

Table statistics from the American Cancer Society's "Cancer Facts & Figures" publications (Atlanta: American Cancer Society, 2009–2013).

1. IOM (Institute of Medicine), *Breast Cancer and the Environment: A life course approach* (Washington, DC: The National Academies Press, 2012), 2.

2. American Cancer Society, "Cancer Facts & Figures 2012," (Atlanta: American Cancer Society, 2012), 4.

3. American Cancer Society, "Breast Cancer Detailed Guide: What are the key statistics about breast cancer?" accessed February 26, 2013, http://www.cancer.org/cancer/breastcancer/detailedguide/breast-cancer-key-statistics.

4. US Cancer Statistics Working Group, *United States Cancer Statistics: 1999–2009 Incidence and Mortality Web-based Report* (Atlanta, Department of Health and Human Services, Centers for Disease Control and Prevention, and National Cancer Institute), 2013, http://apps.nccd.cdc.gov/uscs/.

5. American Cancer Society, *Cancer Facts & Figures 2013* (Atlanta: American Cancer Society, 2013), 9.

The incidence of breast cancer has increased dramatically over recent decades. From 1975 to 2009, desite extensive information on the avoidable causes of breast cancer, its incidence has increased by 24 percent, 11 percent and 29 percent for premenopausal and postmenopausal women respectively. At 142 per 100,000 for white women and 116 for black women, the incidence of breast cancer approaches three times that for lung cancer, which is the second leading cancer diagnosis for white women. Nevertheless, its mortality is sharply decreasing due to improvements in early diagnosis and treatment."[6]

While breast cancer strikes more and more women every year, reader-friendly information on its causes and prevention has still not reached the general public, despite reports and publications by breast cancer activist groups. As detailed in my 2011 Xlibris book, *The National Cancer Institute (NCI) and American Cancer Society (ACS): Criminal Indifference to Cancer Prevention and Conflicts of Interest*, the National Cancer Institute (NCI) and American Cancer Society (ACS) have a vested interest in keeping the public focused on diagnosis, treatment, and basic genetic research, rather than warning of the well-documented risks for developing breast cancer, along with other cancers, in the first place.

The ACS has received contributions of over $100,000 from a wide range of "Excalibur Donors," industries, and companies. Some of them have been responsible for environmental pollution with carcinogens, while others have continued to manufacture and sell products containing carcinogenic ingredients.

Of the members of the ACS board, about half are clinicians, oncologists, surgeons, radiologists, and basic molecular scientists, mostly with close ties to the NCI. Many board members and their institutional colleagues apply for and obtain funding from both the ACS and the NCI. Substantial NCI funds also go to ACS directors who sit on key NCI committees. Although the ACS asks board members to leave the room when the rest of the board discusses their funding proposals, this is just a token formality. In this private club, easy access to funding is one of the "perks," and the board routinely rubber-stamps approvals. A significant amount of ACS research funding

---

6. R. Clapp, G. Howe, and MJ Lefevre, *Environmental and Occupational Causes of Cancer: A Review of Recent Scientific Literature* (University of Massachusetts, 2005).

goes to this extended membership. Frank conflicts of interest are evident in many ACS priorities. These include their policies on mammography, the National Breast Cancer Awareness campaign, and the pesticide and cancer drug industries. These conflicts even extend to the privatization of national cancer policy.

On March 29, 2012, the NCI released a technical thirty-nine-page "Health Professional Version" report on breast cancer prevention.[7] The report was supported by over one hundred scientific references detailing evidence of the "Factors Associated with Increased Risks of Breast Cancer" and of the "Factors Associated with Decreased Risk of Breast Cancer," which are detailed as follows:

Factors Associated With Increased Risk of Breast Cancer
   Hormone therapy
   Ionizing radiation
   Obesity
   Alcohol
   Major inheritance susceptibility

Factors Associated With Decreased Risk of Breast Cancer
   Exercise
   Early pregnancy
   Breast-feeding

Interventions Associated With Decreased Risk of Breast Cancer
   Selective estrogen receptor modulators (SERMs): Benefits
   Selective estrogen receptor modulators (SERMs): Harms
   Aromatase inhibitors or inactivators: Benefits
   Aromatase inhibitors or inactivators: Harms
   Prophylactic mastectomy: Benefits
   Prophylactic mastectomy: Harms
   Prophylactic oophorectomy or ovarian ablation: Benefits
   Prophylactic oophorectomy or ovarian ablation: Harms

---

7. The National Cancer Institute, "Breast Cancer Prevention (PDQ): Health Professional Version," http://cancer.gov/cancertopics/pdq/prevention/breast/healthprofessional/.

Description of Evidence
   Background
   Incidence and mortality
   Etiology and pathogenesis of breast cancer
   Endogenous estrogen
   Genetic mutations

Factors Associated With Increased Risk of Breast Cancer
   Hormone therapy
   Ionizing radiation exposure
   Obesity
   Alcohol

Factors Associated With Decreased Risk of Breast Cancer
   Exercise

Interventions Associated With Decreased Risk of Breast Cancer: Benefits and Harms
   Selective estrogen receptor modulators (SERMs)
   Aromatase inhibition or inactivation
· Prophylactic mastectomy
   Prophylactic oophorectomy
   Fenretinide

Factors of Unproven or Disproven Association
   Abortion
   Oral contraceptives
   Environmental factors
   Diet and vitamins
   Active and passive cigarette smoking
   Statins

One would expect a report like this to hasten attempts to raise awareness about how to avoid such exposures. However, this scientific evidence is in direct contrast to the position of NCI's current director Dr. Harold Varmus.

In astounding ignorance, he has recently claimed that "You can't do experiments to see what causes cancer."[8] Furthermore, and in reckless conflicts of interest, he has consulted with the cancer drug industry, and encouraged his senior staff to do likewise.[9] He has also eliminated price controls on cancer drugs made at the taxpayer expense.[10]

THE ESCALATING INCIDENCE OF BREAST CANCER

	1975	2009	1975–2009
Overall	105	130	23.80%
White	107	132	22%
Black*	94	127	36%
Premenopausal	41	45	11%
Postmenopausal	274	353	29%

THE DECLINING MORTALITY OF BREAST CANCER

	1975	2009	1975–2009
Overall	31	23	-26%
White	32	22	-31%
Black	30	31	3%
Premenopausal	9	5	-44%
Postmenopausal	90	69	-24%

*As reported by Dr. Christine Clark in the July 2012 *Journal of the National Cancer Institute*, the incidence of breast cancer is higher among black than white women before the age of forty but higher among white than black women after the age of forty (The Black/White Crossover).

8. Natalie Angier, *Natural Obsessions: Striving to Unlock the Deepest Secrets of the Cancer Cell* (Boston: Houghton Mifflin Harcourt, 1999), 13.

9. David Willman, "Records of Payments to NIH Staff Sought," *Los Angeles Times,* December 9, 2003. Varmus later appeared before an NIH-convened panel to say his position had changed.

10. Warren E. Leary, "US Gives Up Right to Control Drug Prices," *New York Times,* April 12, 1995.

BREAST CANCER *UN*AWARENESS MONTH

Commenting on the anniversary of the highly publicized October 1994 National Breast Cancer Awareness Month (NBCAM), together with Dr. Jay Gould, director of the Radiation and Public Health Project, I released a statement warning that, "A decade-old, multimillion-dollar deal between National Breast Cancer Awareness Month sponsors and Imperial Chemical Industries (ICI) has produced reckless misinformation on breast cancer."

Zeneca Pharmaceutical, a US subsidiary and recent spinoff of ICI, has been the sole founder of NBCAM since 1985.[11] ICI is one of the largest manufacturers of petrochemical and chlorinated organic products, such as acetochlor and vinyl chloride, and the sole manufacturer of tamoxifen, the world's top-selling cancer drug used to fight breast cancer. Financial sponsorship by Zeneca/ICI gave them editorial control over every leaflet, poster, publication, and commercial produced by NBCAM. NBCAM is promoted by the cancer establishment—the NCI, the ACS, and their corporate sponsors.

The ICI has supported the NCI/ACS blame-the-victim theory of the causes of breast and other cancers. This theory attributes escalating cancer rates to heredity and faulty lifestyle rather than avoidable exposures to industrial carcinogens contaminating air, water, food, consumer products, and the workplace.

RECOGNIZED RISKS

Breast cancer is a complex and heterogeneous group of malignancies that encompass distinct clinical entities, pathologies, and etiologies. Nevertheless, three major classes of overall risk factors for breast cancers have been and still are conventionally recognized. The first is a familial history of breast cancer, particularly early age at onset. The second is reproductive or "estrogen-window" factors: early menarche, nulliparity, late menopause, and exogenous hormones. These include prolonged use of oral contraceptives from an early age, injectable Depo-provera contraceptives, and long-term postmenopausal

---

11. Peter Phillips and Project Censored, "Chemical Corporations Profit Off Breast Cancer," in *Censored 1999: The News That Didn't Make the News*, ed. Peter Phillips (New York: Seven Stories Press, 1999), 34–35.

estrogen replacement therapy (ERT), especially when combined with pro-gestogens, and diethylstilbestrol. The third is a high-fat diet. However, as confirmed by a series of recent case control and cohort studies, evidence for the role of dietary fat per se is at best inconsistent and tenuous. These three risk factors have been incriminated in only 20 to 30 percent of all breast can-cers. Furthermore, they cannot account for the escalating incidence of breast cancer, particularly in postmenopausal women, in the United States and other major industrialized nations. Incidence rates in white women in the United States from 1950 to 1989 increased by 53 percent, or by over 1 percent annu-ally.[12] These trends are real and, in large measure, cannot be explained away by the relatively recent large-scale use of mammography screening. Addi-tionally, these trends are not unique as they are paralleled or even sharply exceeded by those for a wide range of other cancers.

Not one of the heavily funded US and other nutritional studies on the relationship between dietary fat and breast cancer has investigated, let alone even considered, the role of carcinogenic dietary contaminants. However, since the late 1960s it has been known that carcinogenic organochlorine pesticides that concentrate in animal and human fat, such as aldrin, dieldrin, chlordane, and heptachlor, induce breast cancer in rodents.[13] This creates the strong presumption for a causal role of such contaminants in human breast cancer, as the sites of cancer induced by carcinogens in experimental animals and humans are generally similar. Furthermore, DDT induces breast cancer in male rodents by the unrelated carcinogen acetamidophenanthrene. The authors of the latter study concluded that: "Because of their fat-solubility and tendency toward long-term deposition in body fat, particularly in the female breast, and the apparent ability of DDT to promote tumors in the mammary glad of the male rat, such agents might be considered possible contributors to the high incidence of breast cancer among women."[14]

Further evidence for the role of organochlorine carcinogens is provided by findings that DDT and polychlorinated biphenyls (PCBs) concentrate in

---

12. BA Miller, LAG Ries, BF Hankey, CL Kosary, BK Edwards, eds., *Cancer Statistics Review: 1973–1989*, (Bethesda, MD: National Cancer Institute,1992) 1–8.

13. "DDT and associated compounds," *IARC Monograph on Evaluation of Carcinogenic Risks to Humans* 53 (1991): 179–249.

14. JD Scribner and NK Mottet, "DDT acceleration of mammary gland tumors induced in the male Sprague-Dawley rat by 2-acetamidophenanthrene," *Carcinogenesis* 12, no. 2 (1981): 1235–9.

human breast cancer itself in contrast to adjacent non-neoplastic tissue. These organochlorines also concentrate in breasts with cancer in contrast to those with fibrocystic disease. Additionally, the pesticide hexachlorocyclohexane concentrates more in breasts with cancer in contrast to normal breasts. Other and unique supportive evidence comes from reports that, despite increasing fat consumption and decreasing parity, breast cancer mortality in premenopausal Israeli women declined by 30 percent following strong representations by this author[15] and subsequent regulations, opposed by the Israeli cancer establishment, reducing the high levels of hexachlorocyclohexane and DDT in dairy products.[16] The mechanism of action of organochlorine carcinogens in relation to breast cancer probably involves their estrogenic properties, well known for decades, reflecting their potent induction of cytochrome P-450 mixed-function oxidases, stimulation of estrogen metabolism, and binding to human estrogen receptors. Such properties reflect the recent belated recognition of these organochlorines as xeno-estrogens.

Atrazine, a carcinogenic chlorinated triazine, has been and still is one of the most heavily used herbicides in the world. Because of its mobility in soil and its aquatic stability, it is one of the most common carcinogenic pollutants in European and US surface waters, often exceeding the US Health Advisory Level of three parts per billion. Atrazine exerts hormonal effects on the hypothalamic-pituitary-gonadal axis, with marked inhibition of 5-alpha steroid reductase, and induces breast and other reproductive tumors in rats. It has also been incriminated in human ovarian cancer and lymphohematopoietic malignancies. Nevertheless, the role of atrazine in human breast cancer has still not been investigated. Still also ignored is the role of other carcinogenic and estrogenic chlorinated pesticides such as endosulfan and the DDT-contaminated Dicofol.

Estrogens are another important class of dietary contaminants, resulting from their virtually unregulated use as growth-promoting feed additives for cattle, hogs, and poultry. In view of the known carcinogenicity of exogenous estrogens, lifelong exposure to these contaminants is clearly a risk factor for breast cancer, as emphasized by Roy Hertz, the NCI's former leading

---

15. S. S. Epstein, "Carcinogens in Israeli Milk," *Harefuah* 94 (1978): 42–44.

16. J. Westin, "Carcinogens in Israeli Milk: A study in regulatory failure," *International Journal of Health Services* 23 no. 3 (1993): 497–517.

authority on endocrine cancer. Furthermore, estrogens are known to synergize the carcinogenic effects of radiation of the breast, thus possibly further
increasing risks from mammography. Estrogens also synergize the carcinogenic effects in the breast of polynuclear hydrocarbon carcinogens. More
recent concerns on estrogenic dietary contaminants are provided by findings of increased breast cancer risk among women with prenatal exposure
to elevated estrogen levels. This also raises the possibility of similar effects
of prenatal exposure to maternal residues of organochlorine carcinogens.

Proximity of residences to hazardous waste sites has been associated with
major increased risks of breast and other cancers. Most recently, the high
increase in breast cancer incidence and mortality in Connecticut and sub-
urban New York counties, especially Nassau and Suffolk, has been associated
with consumption of milk and water contaminated over the last two decades
with nuclear fission products, the short-lived radioactive iodine and the
long-lived, bone-seeking strontium-90, from the Millstone and Indian Point
civilian nuclear reactors. An additional environmental risk factor in Nassau
and Suffolk counties may reflect past exposure from extensive agricultural use
of carcinogenic soil fumigant pesticides, the organochlorine dichloropropane
and the highly potent organohalogens ethylene dibromide and dibromochlo-
ropropane, all of which induce breast cancer in rodents.

OCCUPATIONAL RISKS

A variety of occupational exposures have been incriminated as risk factors for
breast cancer. Some four million women are currently exposed, often at relatively high levels, to occupational carcinogens. Occupation is thus the single
most important source of involuntary carcinogenic exposures, and responsible
for a wide range of avoidable cancers, particularly breast cancer. Excess incidence and mortality have been reported among women exposed to dioxin—the
most potent known inducer of P-450 enzymes—in a German pesticide plant.

Over one million women, including professional chemists and hair-
dressers, are still exposed to chemicals or processes which have been
incriminated in epidemiological (population) studies. These concerns
have recently been reported in Canadian plastics and automobile workers
involving exposure to formaldehyde, dry cleaning workers exposed to

perchloroethylene, and plastics and rubber workers exposed to organic solvents and benzene. Their risks of breast cancer were more than doubled.

A series of studies exploring the occupational risks of breast cancer were launched in 1995 by James Brophy, Margaret Keith, and a multi-disciplinary team of co-investigators in partnership with the regional cancer centre in Windsor, Ontario, Canada. The work histories for 299 cases of breast cancer were compared to those of another 237 women who had been diagnosed with cancers other than breast or ovarian. The findings, while not statistically strong, revealed a ninefold increase in risk for breast cancer among women who had farmed, particularly among those younger than fifty-five.

"With an expanded research team, Brophy and Keith undertook a subsequent case-control study with improved methods in 2000 to test the farming–breast cancer relationship. The controls were randomly selected from the community. The questionnaire was enhanced to control for the generally accepted breast cancer risk factors, such as reproductive history, and included more detailed questions about the subjects' occupational histories. Analysis revealed the risk of breast cancer almost tripled among women with an occupational history of farming. The risk was also increased for women who worked in farming and subsequently employed in the field of health care or auto-related manufacturing. It was observed that farming tended to be among the earlier jobs worked, often in the teen years. "Because many women who worked in farming began during adolescence, it is plausible that the timing of exposure is of significance in terms of risk."

In order to identify risk factors more specifically, Brophy and Keith and co-investigators launched two follow-up studies: a comprehensive case-control study and a qualitative study, designed to provide them with a deeper understanding of the working conditions for women employed in a few occupations, including farming and automotive manufacturing.[17]

17. JT Brophy, et al., "Occupational histories of cancer patients in a Canadian cancer treatment center and the generated hypothesis regarding breast cancer and farming," *International Journal of Occupational and Environmental Health* 8 (2002): 342–349.

NUMBER OF WOMEN EXPOSED TO OCCUPATIONAL CARCINOGENS

CARCINOGEN	OCCUPATION	APPROXIMATE NUMBERS EXPOSED
Benzene	Solvents; petrochemical synthesis; electrical equipment industries; printing; hand painting, coating, and decorating	143,000
Ethylene oxide	Manufacture of products including detergents, glycol ethers, polyester fibers, and textile chemicals; past major use as hospital sterilant	121,000
Methylene chloride	Solvents; petrochemical manufacturing; electrical equipment; molding and casting machine operators; metal plating; printing; textile; and photography	353,000
Phenylene-diamine dyes	Manufacture and formulation dyes; cosmetologists	200,000

S. S. Epstein, D. Steinman, and S. Levert, *The Breast Cancer Prevention Program* (Hoboken, NJ: Wiley, 1998).

NUCLEAR EMISSIONS

On September 8, 1994, the Cancer Prevention Coalition released a report revealing a significant increase in breast cancer mortality rates among US women living near nuclear facilities.

The report, by Drs. Jay Gould and Ernest Sternglass, was based on a nationwide survey of breast cancer mortality rates in 268 counties within fifty miles of five military facilities and forty-six civilian nuclear power plants. From 1950 to 1989, age-adjusted cancer mortality rates rose from 24 to 26.4 deaths per 100,000 women, a 10 percent increase compared with a 4 percent increase for the nation as a whole.

For the five military plants—Hanford (WA), Idaho (ID), Savannah River (SC), Brookhaven (NY), and Oak Ridge (TN)—the rates of increase were even higher, from 20.7 to 29.2 deaths per 100,000 women, a 41 percent increase. For the seven counties within forty miles of the Oak Ridge plant, the breast cancer mortality rates increased by 39 percent for women living in three downwind counties, in contrast to a 4 percent decrease among women living in four upwind counties. This is consistent with recently published findings of excess cancer mortality rates for both men and women living within a one hundred-mile radius of the Oak Ridge plant.

Based on these data, Dr. Gould concluded, "Nuclear emissions appear linked to increased breast cancer deaths among women living near these facilities. The public has not been informed of its risks."

In a 1991 *Journal of the American Medical Association* article, NCI scientists claimed, "If . . . any excess cancer risk was present in US counties with nuclear facilities, it was too small to be detected with the methods employed."[18] The Gould/Sternglass study raised serious questions about the particular statistical methods by NCI in that they used inappropriate controls based on small populations that were also exposed to nuclear emissions.

SILICONE GEL BREAST IMPLANTS

A September 1994 $4.25 billion settlement to two million women with silicone gel breast implants ignored the risks of developing breast cancer. Of further concern, the Food and Drug Administration (FDA) and the implant industry failed to warn women of serious cancer risks of silicone gel, although they both have known the risks for decades.

A routine FDA inspection in 1987 discovered unpublished Dow Corning studies dating from 1976 onward indicating that silicone gel injection induced malignant tumors in rats. FDA scientists concluded in a 1988 confidential memoranda that: "[W]hile there is no direct proof that silicone causes cancer in humans, there is considerable evidence that it can do so."[19] The memo also recommended that, "a medical alert be issued to warn the

---

18. Seymour Jablon, Zdenek Hrubec, and John D. Boice Jr., "Cancer in populations living near nuclear facilities," *JAMA: the Journal of the American Medical Association* 265, no. 11 (1991): 1403–1408.

19. Sidney M. Wolfe, MD, letter to FDA Commissioner Frank Young, November 9, 1988, http://www.citizen.org/documents/1143.pdf.

public of the possibility of malignancy following long term implant[ation]."[20] However, the FDA's only response was to reassign the concerned scientists. A report in the July 1994 *Journal of the National Cancer Institute* further confirmed gel's carcinogenicity in experiments in mice.[21]

Supporting this experimental evidence, a 1989 confidential FDA report warned: "A survey of the literature indicates numerous case reports of (breast) cancer" long after implantation; that population studies, claimed as proof of safety by industry and plastic surgeons, are too short term and flawed to "negate the potential risk of cancer"; and the "possibility of worsened diagnosis" and prognosis when implanted women developed breast cancer.

At an even higher risk are some 350,000 women with silicone implants wrapped in industrial polyurethane foam to reduce scarring. Polyurethane foam is manufactured from the carcinogenic petrochemical toluene diisocyanate (TDI), which breaks down into another carcinogen, Toluenediamine (TDA). TDI and TDA have also been identified in fresh implants, and TDA has been identified in milk and urine of women with foam implants. It should be further noted that TDA had been removed from hair dyes by the cosmetic industry in 1971 following discovery of its carcinogenicity.

Large-scale use of foam-wrapped implants since the 1980s ignored evidence published two decades before by NCI's leading authority on carcinogenesis, the late Dr. Wilhelm Hueper. His studies showed that foam gradually degrades and induces malignant tumors in rats. He warned: "The definite carcinogenic action of polyurethanes ... provides a warning against indiscriminate use of these plastics in human medical practice." He also noted that carcinogenic effects "might require an induction period of some 30 years or more," as with other carcinogens such as asbestos.[22]

Of still further concern, "there is extensive previously undisclosed documentation of industry's secret knowledge of cancer risks from implants, which were nevertheless marketed with assurances of safety. In fact, Dow Corning's carcinogenicity information on silicone implants is over three

20. Ibid.

21. Michael Potter, Susan Morrison, Francis Wiener, Xiaokui K. Zhang, and Frederick W. Miller, "Induction of Plasmacytomas With Silicone Gel in Genetically Susceptible Strains of Mice," *Journal of the National Cancer Institute* 86, no. 14 (1994): 1058–1065.

22. W. C. Hueper, "Cancer induction by polyurethan and polysilicone plastics," *Journal of the National Cancer Institute* 33, no. 6 (1964): 1005–1027.

decades old." Shortly after foam implants were first marketed on a large scale, a Bristol-Myers subsidiary admitted that: "Degradation products of polyurethane are toxic and in some cases carcinogenic. . . . The breakdown products of the fuzzy implant material may well be carcinogenic. How would anyone defend himself in a malpractice suit if a patient developed a breast malignancy." At a 1985 industry-sponsored conference, a leading plastic surgeon cautioned that "foam could be a time bomb . . . [in view of its] carcinogenic potential. Surgeons should not go on implanting." Following identification of TDA in foam, Bristol-Myers employee warned, ". . . there is pretty solid evidence that [it] is a carcinogen. The question is does PU foam . . . release TDA in the human breast to an extent that causes an unacceptable risk of cancer." Of still further concern is the identification in 1987 of residues of the carcinogenic, sterilizing agent ethylene oxide in foam implants.

Polyurethane implants are carcinogenic-impregnated sponges. The foam gradually disintegrates and releases carcinogens into sensitive breast cells.

To appropriately address this injustice, a medical alert should be sent to all implanted women, with priority for those with foam implants. This should be followed by offers to remove the implants of concerned women at industry's expense, quite apart from the recent $4.25 billion dollar settlement. This should also be followed by comprehensive surveillance of all implanted women.

TAMOXIFEN AND EVISTA

Tamoxifen (Nolvadex) and evista (Raloxifene) are anti-estrogenic hormonal drugs, known as selective estrogen receptor modulators (SERMS). Both drugs have been shown in large-scale clinical trials to reduce the risk of breast cancer, especially in postmenopausal women at high risk. Notably, these are women over the age of sixty with a family history of breast cancer. While tamoxifen is more effective, evista may be less risky, particularly with regard to the lower incidence of complications, notably uterine cancer, blood clots, and cataracts. Evista has also been shown to prevent and treat osteoporosis.

Based on the results of the 2010 Study of Tamoxifen and Raloxifene

(STAR) trial, tamoxifen has been shown to be much more effective than evista in reducing the risks and recurrence of breast cancer.[23]

According to WebMD Health News, the costs of both drugs are about $8,400 for five years of prevention, in comparison with costs from $50,000 to $120,000 for treating one early breast cancer case.[24]

GENETIC RISKS

Breast cancer is the most common cancer in women. Less than 5 percent of breast cancer patients have a familial risk of cancer due to inherited mutations in their BRCA1 or BRCA2 genes.

Overall, about 2 percent of breast cancer cases are directly related to these genes which are highly sensitive to mammography radiation. Women who carry either of them have about a 16 percent chance of developing breast cancer.

THE WAR AGAINST CANCER

The launching of President Nixon's 1971 war against cancer provided the ACS with a well-exploited opportunity to pursue its own myopic and self-interested agenda. ACS conflicts of interest are extensive but still unrecognized by the public. Meanwhile, the ACS continues to ignore a wide range of industrial carcinogens in water, air, food, the workplace, and in mainstream household, cosmetics, and personal care products.

ACS strategies remain based on two myths: first, that there has been dramatic progress in the treatment and cure of cancer, and second, that any increase in the incidence and mortality of cancer is due to aging of the population and smoking, while denying any significant role for involuntary exposures to industrial and other carcinogens.

As the world's largest nonreligious "charity," with powerful allies in the private and public sectors, ACS policies and priorities remain unchanged.

---

23. National Cancer Institute, "The Study of Tamoxifen and Raloxifene (STAR): Questions and Answers," updated April 19, 2010, http://www.cancer.gov/newscenter/qa/2006/starresultsqandA.

24. Charlene Laino, "Tamoxifen, Evista Prevent Breast Cancer," WebMD.com, April 20, 2010, http://www.webmd.com/breast-cancer/news/20100420/tamoxifen-evista-preent-breast-cancer.

Despite periodic protest, threats of boycotts, and questions concerning its finances, the ACS leadership responds with powerful public relations campaigns reflecting denial and manipulated information, while pillorying its opponents with scientific McCarthyism.

The verdict is unassailable. The ACS bears a major decades-long responsibility for losing the winnable war against cancer. Reforming the ACS is, in principle, relatively easy and directly achievable. Boycott the ACS. Instead, give your charitable contributions to public interest and environmental groups involved in cancer prevention.

Such a boycott is well overdue and will send the only message this "charity" can no longer ignore.

THE CANCER DRUG INDUSTRY

The intimate association between the ACS and the cancer drug industry, with annual sales of over $12 billion, is further illustrated by the unbridled aggression which the ACS has directed at its critics.

Just as Senator Joseph McCarthy had his "black list" of suspected communists and Richard Nixon his environmental activist "enemies list," so too, the ACS maintains a "Committee on Unproven Methods of Cancer Management"[25] which periodically "reviews" unorthodox or alternative therapies. This committee is comprised of "volunteer health care professionals," carefully selected proponents of orthodox, expensive, and usually toxic drugs patented by major pharmaceutical companies, and opponents of alternative or "unproven" therapies which are generally cheap, nonpatentable, and minimally toxic.

Periodically, the committee updates its statements on "unproven methods," which are then widely disseminated to clinicians, cheerleader science writers, and the public. Once a clinician or oncologist becomes associated with "unproven methods," he or she is blackballed by the cancer establishment. Funding for the accused "quack" becomes inaccessible, followed by systematic harassment.

---

25. William T. Jarvis, "Cancer Quackery," National Council Against Health Fraud, http://ncahf.org/articles/c-d/caquackery.html. The Committee's name was changed in 1995 to the "Subcommittee on Alternative and Complementary Methods of Cancer Management."

The highly biased ACS witch-hunts against alternative practitioners is in striking contrast to its extravagant and uncritical endorsement of conventional toxic chemotherapy, despite the absence of any objective evidence of improved survival rates or reduced mortality following chemotherapy for all but some relatively rare cancers.

In response to pressure from People Against Cancer, a grassroots group of cancer patients disillusioned with conventional cancer therapy, in 1986 some forty members of Congress requested the Office of Technology Assessment (OTA), a congressional think tank, to evaluate available information on alternative innovative therapies. While initially resistant, the OTA eventually published a September 1990 report that identified some two hundred promising studies on alternative therapies. The OTA concluded that the NCI had "mandated responsibility to pursue this information and facilitate examination of widely used 'unconventional cancer treatments' for therapeutic potential."[26]

Yet the ACS and NCI remained resistant, if not frankly hostile, to the OTA's recommendations. In the January 1991 issue of its *Cancer Journal for Clinicians,* the ACS referred to the Hoxsey therapy, a nontoxic combination of herb extracts developed in the 1940s by populist Harry Hoxsey, as a "worthless tonic for cancer." However, a detailed critique of Hoxsey's treatment by Dr. Patricia Spain Ward, a leading contributor to the OTA report, concluded just the opposite: "More recent literature leaves no doubt that Hoxsey's formula does indeed contain many plant substances of marked therapeutic activity."[27]

This is not the first time that the Society's charges of quackery have been called into question or discredited. A growing number of other innovative therapies originally attacked by the ACS have recently found less disfavor and even acceptance. These include hyperthermia, tumor necrosis factor (originally called Coley's toxin), hydrazine sulfate, and Burzynski's antineoplastons. Well over one hundred promising alternative nonpatented and nontoxic therapies have been identified. Clearly, such treatments merit clinical testing and evaluation, using similar statistical techniques and criteria

---

26. United States Congress OTA, *Unconventional Cancer Treatments* (Washington, DC: US Government Printing Office, 1990).

27. R. W. Moss, *Questioning Chemotherapy* (Brooklyn, NY: Equinox Press, 1995).

as established for conventional chemotherapy. However, while the FDA has approved approximately forty patented drugs for cancer treatment, it has still not approved a single nonpatented alternative drug.

Subsequent events have further isolated the ACS in its fixation on "orthodox treatments." Bypassing the ACS and NCI, the National Institutes of Health opened a new Office of Alternative Medicine for the investigation of unconventional treatment of cancer and other diseases in June 1992. Leading proponents of conventional therapy were invited to participate. The ACS refused. The NCI grudgingly and nominally participated while actively attacking alternative therapy with its widely circulated *Cancer Information Services*. Meanwhile, the NCI's police partner, the FDA, used its enforcement authority against distributors and practitioners of innovative and nontoxic therapies.

In an interesting development, the Washington, DC, Center for Mind-Body Medicine held a two-day conference on Comprehensive Cancer Care: Integrating Complementary and Alternative Therapies. According to Dr. James Gordon, former president of the Center and chair of the Program Advisory Council of the NIH Office of Alternative Medicine,[28] the object of the conference was to bring together practitioners of mainstream and alternative medicine, together with cancer patients and high-ranking officials of the ACS and NCI. Dr. Gordon warned alternative practitioners that "they're going to need to get more rigorous with their work—to be accepted by the mainstream community."[29] However, no such warning was directed at the highly questionable claims of the NCI and ACS for the efficacy of conventional cancer chemotherapy. As significantly, criticism of the establishment's minimalistic priority for cancer prevention was effectively discouraged.

Not surprising is the conclusion "that there has been no progress in preventing the disease,"[30] despite US expenditure of over $1 billion on breast cancer over the last two decades. More surprising, however, is the persisting

---

28. Now the National Center for Complementary and Alternative Medicine (NCCAM).

29. L. Castelucci, "Practitioners seek common ground in unconventional forum." *Journal of the National Cancer Institute* 90: 136–137, 1998.

30. "Prospects for Breast Cancer Remain Same, Study Finds," *The Washington Post*, December 12, 1991. Quote from Richard Linster, General Account Office Director of Planning and Reporting.

failure of the US cancer establishment—the NCI and the ACS—to have recognized and investigated longstanding evidence on the role of a wide range of avoidable environmental and occupational risk factors for breast cancer besides for a wide range of other cancers. Their recognition should result in the belated development of public health policies directed to primary prevention of breast and other cancers, and should also further reinforce recommendations for major reforms in the priorities and leadership of the cancer establishment.

SUSAN G. KOMEN'S CONFLICTS OF INTEREST, 2012

As announced in the *New York Times* on February 2, 2012, the Susan G. Komen for the Cure Foundation announced a decision to terminate its decades-long partnership and $700,000 funding of Planned Parenthood, which provides abortion services to affiliates in nationwide clinics. The Komen Foundation also provides breast cancer screening and education to low-income women.

Faced with prompt nationwide criticisms, Nancy Brinker, Komen's chief executive, held a news conference attempting to deny that this decision had anything to do with politics, particularly offending anti-abortion activists and Republican presidential candidates. She also promptly restored relationship with Planned Parenthood.

As noted in the February 3, 2012 issue of the *Cancer Letter*, Brinker's message on the Komen website enthused, "We have come a long way in our fight. When we started, the five-year survival rate was just 74 percent when breast cancer was diagnosed before it spread beyond the breast. Today, that survival rate is 98 percent . . . We are so close to creating a world without breast cancer. The science is there."[31] However, there is no basis for this extravagant claim, as first year survival rates provide little or no basis for any longer survival.

---

31. Paul Goldberg, "The Pink Machine Sputters, Goes In Reverse: Komen Funding Decision Sparks Outrage," *The Cancer Letter* 38 no. 5 (February 3, 2012).

CHAPTER 2

Avoidable Causes of Breast Cancer

The causes of breast cancer are all around us. The good news is, many of them are avoidable. Consider reducing your exposure to the following factors in order to reduce your risk.

LIFESTYLE

- Cosmetics and personal care products containing hormonal (endocrine disruptive) ingredients, such as bisphenol-A, parabens, and phthalates, and aluminum chloride anti-perspirants
- Dark hair dyes, with early and prolonged use
- Alcohol, with early and excessive use
- Tobacco smoking (active or passive), with early and excessive use
- Inactivity: regular exercise reduces risks by up to 30 percent
- Obesity: weight loss after age eighteen can reduce risks by up to 50 percent
- Shift work, particularly at night
- Meat from cattle implanted with natural or synthetic sex hormones
- Genetically-engineered (rBGH) milk contaminated with a growth factor (IGF-1), which increases risks of breast cancer by up to sevenfold

ENVIRONMENTAL/OCCUPATIONAL

- Ionizing radiation, the longest-known environmental cause of breast cancer
- Premenopausal exposure to tobacco smoke
- Exposure to carcinogenic household products
- Occupational exposure to a wide range of carcinogens (including: benzene, ethylene oxide, formaldehyde, carbon tetrachloride, dichloromethane, and vinyl chloride)

- Proximity of residence to petrochemical and operating nuclear reactors, and superfund hazardous waste sites
- Atrazine-contaminated drinking water
- Domestic exposure to EMF (electromagnetic field) radiation from electric blankets "Endocrine disruptors," also known as synthetic estrogens, which mimic the actions of estrogens, found in many pesticides, fuels, plastics, detergents, and prescription drugs[32]
- Dietary exposure to the estrogenic effects of cadmium pollutants
- Diets high in animal and dairy fats contaminated with carcinogenic, estrogenic, and endocrine disruptive pollutants
- Workplace exposure to a wide range of carcinogens

MEDICAL

- Induced abortion[33]
- Nulliparity or delayed parity
- Obesity
- No breast feeding
- Mammography, with early and repeated exposures (However, it can be justified for pre-menopausal women with close relatives diagnosed with breast cancer under the age of fifty.)
- Diagnostic radiation, particularly computerized axial tomography (CAT) breast scans[34]
- Oral contraceptives (the "Pill"), with early and prolonged use[35]
- Estrogen replacement therapy (ERT), with high doses and prolonged use
- Nonhormonal prescription drugs, such as diazepam tranquilizers, and anti-hypertensives

32. R. Clapp, G. Howe, and M. J. Lefevre, *Environmental and Occupational Causes of Cancer: A Review of Recent Scientific Literature* (University of Massachusetts, 2005).

33. Evidence is equivocal, and has been challenged by the World Health Organization in Fact Sheet No. 240, June 2000.

34. A. Pijpe et al., "Exposure to diagnostic radiation and risk of breast cancer among carriers of BRCA1/2 mutations: retrospective cohort study (GENE-RAD-RISK)," *BMJ* 345 (2012): e5660.

35. Collaborative Group on Hormonal Factors in Breast Cancer, "Breast cancer and hormonal contraceptives: collaborative reanalysis of individual data on 53,297 women with breast cancer and 100,239 women without breast cancer from 54 epidemiological studies," *Lancet* 347, no. 9017 (1996):1713–1727.

- Silicone gel breast implants, especially those wrapped in polyurethane foam
- Repeated X-radiation of the chest or neck, especially for diagnosis in children
- Human growth hormone (HGH), anti-aging medication
- Ionizing radiation from diagnostic procedures, particularly fluoroscopy
- Diethylstilbestrol (DES), a synthetic estrogenic hormone prescribed to pregnant women, and designed to prevent miscarriage

HORMONAL AND INDUSTRIAL RISKS OF BREAST CANCER

	IARC*	NTP**
Hormones (pharmaceutical and personal care products)		
Hormone replacement therapy and oral contraceptives	Yes	Yes
Diethylstilbestrol	Yes	Yes
Estrogens in personal care products	Yes	Yes
Endocrine-Disruptive Ingredients		
Dioxins	Yes	Yes
Dichlorodiphenyltrichloroethane (DDT)		Yes
Dichlorodiphenyldichloroethylene (DDE)		Yes
Tobacco smoke (active and passive exposures)	Yes	Yes
Metals	Yes	Yes
Industrial Chemicals		
Benzene	Yes	Yes
Vinyl Chloride	Yes	Yes
Ethylene oxide	Yes	Yes

*International Agency for Research on Cancer
**National Toxicology Program

Further concerns include a wide range of the following avoidable causes of breast cancer:

- **Since the 1950s scientific evidence has incriminated chlorinated organic pesticides as breast cancer risk factors** because of their carcinogenicity, estrogenic effects, and accumulation in body fat, particularly the breast.

- **The unregulated use of growth promoting hormonal cattle feed additives has resulted in near universal contamination of meat products.** This results in life-long exposure to carcinogenic estrogens and poses a major avoidable risk of breast cancer.

- **Where you work may increase your breast cancer risks.** Excess breast cancers were found in the 1970s in women working with vinyl chloride. There is similar evidence among petrochemical and electrical workers. Despite more women working in such industries, the NCI recently admitted that it has still not investigated these risks among working women.

- **Where you live may increase risks of breast cancer.** Based on a review of twenty-one New Jersey counties,[36] and more recently 339 nationwide counties,[37] statistically significant associations were found between excess breast cancer mortality and residence in counties where hazardous waste sites are located.

- **Living near a nuclear facility increases your chances of dying from breast cancer.** Based on a nationwide survey of 268 counties within fifty miles of fifty-one military and civilian nuclear reactors, CPC member Dr. Jay Gould, showed that breast cancer mortality in these "nuclear counties" has increased at ten times the national rate from 1950 to 1989. Counties near military reactors, such as Hanford, Oak Ridge, and Savannah River, have registered the greatest increases, ranging from 27 to 200 percent. Dr. Gould charged NCI with "misrepresentation of such findings."[38]

- **Premenopausal mammography increases your risk of breast cancer.** Increases in breast cancer incidence and mortality have been consistently reported following repeated mammography in

---

36. G.R. Najem and T.W. Greer, "Female reproductive organs and breast cancer mortality in New Jersey counties and the relationship with certain environmental variables," *Preventive Medicine* 14 no. 5 (September 1985):620–35.

37. Sandra Steingraber, *Living Downstream* (Cambridge, MA: Da Capo Press, 2010), 70.

38. Jay Gould, *The Enemy Within* (New York: Four Walls Eight Windows, 1996).

younger women in six randomized controlled clinical trials over the last decade. Based on this evidence, the NCI has recently withdrawn recommendations for premenopausal mammography. The ACS, with financial support from DuPont and General Electric (both heavily invested in mammography equipment), and self-interested radiologists are still promoting this dangerous practice.

- **Breast implants, particularly polyurethane foam, pose serious risks of breast cancer.** Evidence on the carcinogenicity of polyurethane foam dates back to the early 1960s. One breakdown product of polyurethane is 2,4-toluenediamine which was removed from hair dyes in 1971 following discovery of its carcinogenicity. Frank admission of these risks are found in internal NCI, FDA and industry documents.

- **The tamoxifen "chemoprevention" trial is a travesty!** Since 1992, the cancer establishment recruited sixteen thousand healthy women in a tamoxifen "chemoprevention" trial. NCI and ACS claimed, in their patient consent forms, that tamoxifen could substantially reduce breast cancer risks, while trivializing risks of drug complications. There is strong evidence of tamoxifen's toxicity, including high risks of uterine, gastrointestinal, and fatal liver cancer.[39] This trial was scientifically and ethically reckless, and participating institutions and clinicians are still at risk of future malpractice claims.

- Participation in the reckless 1972 NCI/ACS high dose mammography experiments increased breast cancer risks for the four hundred thousand women involved.[40]

- Genetically engineered (rBGH) milk increases risks of breast cancer due to its increased levels of insulin-like growth.[41]

- Dosing aged monkeys with insulin-like growth factor (IGF-1) induced a highly significant increase in breast size, and strong stimulatory effects in breast cells. The authors warned of risks of breast cancer from

39. Avi Barbasch, "Breast Cancer Prevention: Tamoxifen and Dietary Considerations," in *Genetic Susceptibility to Breast and Ovarian Cancer: Assessment, Counseling, and Testing Guidelines* (Bethesda, MD: American College of Medical Genetics), 1999.

40. Herbert Seidman et al., "Survival Experience in the Breast Cancer Detection and Demonstration Project," *CA: A Cancer Journal for Clinicians* 37 no.5, Sept/Oct 1987, 258-90. From 1972-1975, more than 280,000 women were enrolled in the project.

41. Epstein, S.S. *What's In Your Milk?* Trafford Publishing, 2006.

treating postmenopausal women with IGF-1.

- In a prospective study of three hundred healthy nurses, those with elevated IGF-1 blood levels were strongly associated with up to a sevenfold risk of pre-menopausal breast cancer.

DANGERS OF OBESITY[42]

- A 1977 study in *Preventive Medicine* found that breast cancer risk in obese postmenopausal women was about 50 percent greater than in the nonobese.
- A 1977 Netherlands report in *Cancer* showed that the overall risk of postmenopausal breast cancer increases in proportion to womens' weight. Furthermore, the more overweight the woman, the more serious the cancer.
- In 1978, a report in *Preventive Medicine* revealed that Japanese women over fifty and at least 5 percent above the national average weight were at a significantly increased risk. A 1978 Canadian report in the *American Journal of Epidemiology* also found an excess breast cancer rate among heavier menopausal women.
- A large-scale 1979 ACS study in the *Journal of Chronic Disease* reported that breast cancer mortality was 50 percent greater in very obese women compared with those carrying less excess weight.
- A 1979 study in the *Journal of the National Cancer Institute* confirmed that breast cancer risks increased progressively with weight.
- A 1980 study in the *American Journal of Epidemiology* found the heaviest women had an almost 40 percent increased risk compared with the lightest.
- A 1983 study in the *American Journal of Epidemiology* showed that any degree of obesity was associated with a 50 percent increase in risk.
- A 1988 study of Chinese women, published in *Cancer Research,* found that "high average body weight" was associated with breast cancer risk, especially among women over age sixty.
- A 1994 Netherlands report in the *British Journal of Cancer* found

---

42. Epstein, Steinman, and Levert, *The Breast Cancer Prevention Program* (Hoboken, NJ: Wiley 1998).

PRESIDENT OBAMA'S CANCER PANEL: REDUCING ENVIRONMENTAL AND OCCUPATIONAL LINKS WITH BREAST CANCER AND WHAT WE CAN DO NOW, 2008–2009

Category	Carcinogenic Agent	Sources/Uses	Strong	Suspected
Environmental Tobacco Smoke	Over 50 carcinogens	Also known as passive or environmental tobacco smoke	Yes	
Pesticides	Herbicides, Fungicides, Insecticides	Used for preventing, destroying, repelling, or mitigating pests, and also as plant regulators, defoliants, or desiccants.		Yes
Petrochemical and Combustion By-Products	Motor Vehicle Exhaust, Polycyclic Aromatic Hydrocarbons, Soot, Dioxins	Petrochemicals derived from natural gas or petroleum and used to produce other chemicals, including pesticides, plastics, and dyes.		Yes
Radiation	Ionizing	Several types of particles and X-rays given off by radioactive material, high-voltage equipment and nuclear reactors.	Yes	
Radiation	Non-ionizing	Microwaves and Electromagnetic frequencies, including radio waves and extremely low-frequency electromagnetic		Yes
Reactive Chemicals	Ethylene Oxide	Used as a sterilant, disinfectant, and pesticide. Also used as a raw ingredient in making resins, films, and antifreeze.		Yes
Hormone	Diethystilbestrol	A synthetic estrogen prescribed to pregnant women, designed to prevent miscarriage at risk of breast cancer.	Yes	
Solvents	PCBs (Polychlorinated Biphenyls), Bisphenol-A	Used as coolants and lubricants in transformers, capacitors, and other electronic equipment		Yes

Epstein, Steinman, and Levert, *The Breast Cancer Prevention Program* (Hoboken, NJ: Wiley, 1998).

that risk of breast cancer increased 90 percent among the heaviest women.

- A 1996 study on Asian Americans in the *Journal of the National Cancer Institute,* reported twice the risk among the heaviest rather than the lightest women. "Women in their fifties . . . with a recent gain of more than 10 pounds had three times the risk."

DANGERS OF HAIR DYES[43]

- A 1976 study in the *New York State Journal of Medicine* reported that eighty-seven of one hundred breast cancer patients had been long-term hair dye users.
- A 1977 United Kingdom study in the *British Medical Journal* found an increased risk among hair dye users over the age of fifty whose first pregnancy had occurred after the age of thirty.
- A 1979 United States study in the *Journal of the National Cancer Institute* found a significant relationship between frequency and duration of hair dye use and breast cancer. The relation was even stronger for women with a "low natural risk for breast cancer." Women at greatest risk were fifty to seventy-nine years old.
- Another 1979 study in *The Lancet* reported excess breast cancers among American women who had used hair dyes for at least twenty-one years. Again, one of the key factors in this increased risk was long-term use.
- A well-controlled 1980 study reported in the *Journal of the National Cancer Institute* found that women who dyed their hair to change its color, in contrast to just masking grayness, were at threefold risk. These risks were even greater for women aged forty to fifty, and with a past history of benign breast disease, and for women aged forty to forty-nine.

43. S. S. Epstein, and R. Fitzgerald, *Healthy Beauty* (Dallas, TX: BenBella Books, 2009).

DANGERS OF HORMONAL CONTRACEPTIVES[44]

- In 1977, a study published in *Cancer* found that the risk of breast cancer increased after two to four years of oral contraceptive (the Pill) use, and further increased in women with a history of benign breast disease and who had not had a full-term pregnancy.

- A 1981 study published in the *British Journal of Cancer* reported a nearly fourfold increased risk in women under the age of thirty-three who had used oral contraceptives for eight years before their first pregnancy.

- In 1982, the *American Journal of Epidemiology* announced that women aged thirty-five to fifty-four who at any time used the Pill before their first childbirth tripled their risk of breast cancer. The longer they had used oral contraceptives, the more their risk increased.

- In 1986, a joint study from Sweden and Norway published in *The Lancet* revealed that women under the age of forty-five doubled their risk if they used the Pill for more than seven years before having their first child.

- A 1987 study published in the *British Journal of Cancer* reported that women under the age of forty-five who had used the Pill for over four years before their first full-term pregnancy more than doubled their risk.

- A 1988 study from Slovenia published in *Neoplasia* reported that the overall risk of breast cancer increased significantly with duration of use, particularly for seven or more years. This risk increased to more than sevenfold in women with a family history.

- In 1988, the "Cancer and Steroid Hormone Study" published in the journal *Contraception* revealed that women who had used the Pill for eight years or more, had never given birth, and had begun menstruating before the age of thirteen were all at increased risk for developing breast cancer before the age of forty-five. This risk was nearly threefold for eight to eleven years of use, and twelvefold for twelve or more years of use.

---

44. Epstein, Steinman, and Levert, *The Breast Cancer Prevention Program* (Hoboken, NJ: Wiley 1998).

- In 1989, Swedish investigators reported to the *Journal of the National Cancer Institute* that using the Pill at a young age increases the risk of breast cancer: "Both the duration of oral contraceptive use before twenty-five years of age and commencement of oral contraceptive use at a young age were associated with a significant increase in the risk of breast cancer."[45]

- In 1990, an analysis of some thirty-two studies published in the journal *Cancer* revealed a "statistically positive trend in the risk of premenopausal breast cancer for women exposed to OCs for longer duration." This risk was predominant among women who used oral contraceptives for at least four years before their first full-term pregnancy.

- In 1991, an eleven-nation study published in *Contraception* demonstrated a "small increase" in the risk of breast cancer in recent and current users. This risk increased with duration of use.

- In 1994, a large, well-controlled study published in the *Journal of the National Cancer Institute* reported a "small increased risk of breast cancer associated with long duration of oral contraceptive use." The increase in risk was about 30 percent, but increased to 70 percent "particularly among women aged 35 years or younger." A thirty-old-woman, then, increased her risk from 1 in 2,525 to 1 in 764.

- In 1995, a National Cancer Institute study reported a definite link between the length of time oral contraceptives are used and the risk of breast cancer. A few months of use could increase a woman's risk by 30 percent. A more than twofold risk was found with ten years of use or longer. The same study also showed that oral contraceptive use was associated with cancer in its most advanced stages at diagnosis in women under the age of thirty-five.

- According to a meta-analysis published in *Mayo Clinic Proceedings* in 2006, "The use of oral contraceptives (OC) is associated with an increased risk of premenopausal breast cancer."[46] This association was greatest for women who used OCs for four or more years before their first full term pregnancy.

---

45. HÅkan Olsson et al., "Early oral contraceptive use and breast cancer among premenopausal women: Final report from a study in southern Sweden," *JNCI J Natl Cancer Inst.* 81 no. 13 (1989): 1000–1004.

46. C. Kahlenborn, et al., "Oral contraceptive use as a risk factor for premenopausal breast cancer: a meta-analysis," *Mayo Clin Proc.* 81 (2006): 1290–1302.

DANGERS OF ESTROGEN REPLACEMENT THERAPY (ERT)[47]

- In 1991, an *American Journal of Epidemiology* article cited eight major studies demonstrating increased risks of breast cancer, ranging from 20 to 80 percent, among women using ERT for extended periods.
- In 1991, pooled results from sixteen previous studies, published in the *Journal of the American Medical Association*, reported that women who used ERT for over fifteen years increased their risk of breast cancer by up to 30 percent. Among women reporting a family history of breast cancer, the risks were tenfold higher.
- Another pooled analysis similarly found that women who used ERT for at least eight years had a 25 to 30 percent increased risk.
- In 1995, the "Harvard Nurses' Health Study" confirmed an increased risk of 30 to 70 percent for women using ERT. This risk increased with cumulative use after five years.
- A large-scale study based on sixty thousand postmenopausal women, and published in the June 1997 *New England Journal of Medicine*, reported that the use of ERT for over ten years increased breast cancer deaths by 43 percent.

DANGERS OF ENDOCRINE DISRUPTIVE OR HORMONAL INGREDIENTS IN COSMETICS AND PERSONAL CARE PRODUCTS

Endocrine disruptive ingredients are a large group of synthetic hormonal chemicals known as xenoestrogens, which are common ingredients in cosmetics and personal care products. As detailed in my 2009 book, *Healthy Beauty* (BenBella), these include over twenty ingredients, preservatives such as parabens, detergents such as EDTA, and solvents such as bisphenol-A.

---

47. Epstein, Steinman, and Levert, *The Breast Cancer Prevention Program* (Hoboken, NJ: Wiley 1998).

CARCINOGENIC AND HORMONAL DANGERS OF COSMETICS

Cosmetic Ingredient	Breast Carcinogen	Hormonal Compound	Uses
Butadiene	Yes		In shaving creams, hair mousse, hair styling gels and some high-SPF sunscreens
Dioxane	Yes		Contaminant in products containing ethoxylate ingredients
Benzene	Yes		An impurity of toluene, found in some nail polish
Bisphenol A		Yes	Cosmetics containers/packaging
Ethosylates (contaminated with dioxane	Yes		Shampoos, body wash, children's bath products and sudsing products
Ethylene oxide	Yes		Fragrance
Heavy metals		Yes	Cadmium and lead may be present in lipsticks and face paints, and mercury in masacras
Synthetic musks		Yes	Fragrance
Nitrosamines			Contaminant present in diethoanolamine or triethanolamine
Nonylphenol		Yes	Lotions
Parabens		Yes	Antifungal preservative and antimicrobial in creams, lotions, and ointments
Petrolatum (contaminated with polycyclic aromatic hydrocarbons)	Yes	Yes	Ingredient in petroleum jelly, lipsticks, baby lotions and oils
Phthalates		Yes	Nail polish, fragrance, cosmetics, containers/packaging
Titanium dioxide		Yes	Sunscreens and mineral makeup. Nanoparticles of titanium dioxide are of particular concern

| Triclosan | | Yes | Antibacterial used in soaps, toothpaste, mouthwash, and other personal care products |
| Urethane | Yes | | Hair care products, sunscreens, nail polish, mascara, foundation |

"What is the Connection Between Cosmetics and Breast Cancer?," Breast Cancer Fund, October 10, 2007.

DANGERS OF DIAGNOSTIC AND THERAPEUTIC RADIATION[48]

- In 1965, a study in the *British Journal of Cancer* reported increased cancer rates after repeated and prolonged exposure to X-rays taken to monitor the progress of tuberculosis treatment. Each examination exposed the breast by up to 8 rads (radiation absorbed dose), and patients typically received one hundred examinations or more.

- In 1971, the *Journal of the American Medical Association* reported excess breast cancers in adults who as children had received irradiation to the thymus gland. From the 1920s until 1955, doctors routinely used chest X-rays to diagnose an allegedly abnormal enlargement of the gland in young children.

- Reports in the *Canadian Medical Association Journal, Radiology*, and the *Journal of the National Cancer Institute* from 1973 to 1977 confirmed an excess of breast cancers among women with past history of repeated chest radiation.

- In 1989, a small study in the *Journal of the National Cancer Institute* reported excess breast cancers among women who had been treated with X-rays for spinal curvature as children. These women had received an average breast dose of 13 rads at an average age of twelve.

- Another 1989 study in *The Lancet* found excess breast cancer rates in women whose doctors treated fungal infections of their scalps with radiation and whose breasts were exposed to less than 2 rads.

---

48. Epstein, Steinman, and Levert, *The Breast Cancer Prevention Program* (Hoboken, NJ: Wiley, 1998).

- In 1996, the *New England Journal of Medicine* published a study showing that the breast cancer risk is much higher than normal among women treated with radiation for childhood Hodgkin's disease.

- Based on a detailed review of these and a wide range of other such studies, Dr. John Gofman, a leading international authority on medical radiation, published his analysis in a startling book, *Preventing Breast Cancer*. Gofman warned that past medical radiation is probably the single most important cause of the modern breast cancer epidemic. An editorial in the *Journal of the American Medical Association* attacked this conclusion as "incredible,"[49] as accusation vigorously and successfully challenged by Gofman in a later issue of the same journal.[50]

- The October 26, 2011 *New York Times* article "More Questions About Mammograms," based on an analysis of the *Archive of Internal Medicine*, concluded that the "vast majority" of women "do not benefit" from mammography—"probably because they have slow-growing cancers that would never have killed them or could have been treated at an early stage."[51]

- These warnings were further detailed in a December 26, 2011 *CounterPunch* article on "The Dangers of CT Scans: The Leading Cause of Breast Cancer." Published by the National Academy's Institute of Medicine, the article warned that "the large radiation dose delivered by CT scans is the foremost identifiable cause of breast cancer."[52]

- As reported in June 2012 by Dr. Moskowitz, a biostatistician at the Memorial Sloan-Kettering Cancer Center in New York, "women who received chest radiation to treat childhood cancer had a high risk of developing breast cancers as an adult."[53]

49. Andrew A Skolnick, "Claim that Medical X-Rays Caused Most US Breast Cancers Found Indredible," *Journal of the American Medical Association* 274 no. 5 (1995), 367–8.

50. John W Gofman, "X-Rays and Breast Cancer," *JAMA* 274 no. 22 (1995), 1762.

51. "More Questions About Mammograms," *The New York Times*, October 26 2011, http://www.nytimes.com/2011/10/27/opinion/more-questions-about-mammograms.html?_r=0.

52. John LaForge, "The Dangers of CT Scans: The Leading Cause of Breast Cancer," *CounterPunch*, December 26 2011, http://www.counterpunch.org/2011/12/26/the-leading-cause-of-breast-cancer/.

53. Andrew Pollack, "A Drug for Advanced Melanoma is Found to Prolong Patients' Lives," *The New York Times*, June 4 2012. <http://www.nytimes.com/2012/06/04/health/glaxosmithkline-melanoma-drug-prolongs-patients-lives.html>.

DANGERS OF PESTICIDES[54]

- A 1976 World Health Organization study of Brazilian women found that the industrial pollutants, polychlorinated biphenyls (PCBs) and the pesticide DDT, selectively concentrate in breast cancer in contrast with nearby noncancerous tissues. Other pesticides, either carcinogenic and/or estrogenic to the breast (benzene hexachloride, dieldrin, and heptachlor epoxide), demonstrated "more or less the same tendency."

- A small 1982 study reported high concentrations of DDT and benzene hexachloride in breast cancers compared to adjacent normal breast tissue.

- Higher levels of benzene hexachloride were found in breast cancers compared to normal breast tissues in a well-controlled 1990 study. Women with the highest levels were at a nearly eleven times greater risk of breast cancer.

- A 1992 study found that concentrations of PCBs and DDE, a breakdown product of DDT, were up to 60 percent higher in tissues of women with cancer compared to those with benign breast disease.

- A 1993 study reported that women with the highest blood levels of DDE were at four times great risk for breast cancer compared to those with the lowest levels.

- In 1994, Canadian researchers reported that concentrations of a wide range of carcinogenic and pseudoestrogenic pesticides and industrial pollutants were higher in the fat and blood of women with estrogen-sensitive breast cancers than in healthy women.

- A "strong, positive association between DDE (a derivative of DDT) and breast cancer in Caucasian and African-American [women]" was reported in a 1994 study, supporting a three- to fourfold increase among Caucasians with the highest exposures.

DANGERS OF DIETARY EXPOSURE TO CADMIUM

Cadmium is well known as an industrial pollutant from the combustion of

---

54. Epstein, Steinman, and Levert, *The Breast Cancer Prevention Program.*

fossil fuels and sewage sludge. Additional exposures result from the use of cadmium as fertilizer.

A Swedish study, published by the American Association for Cancer Research on March 15, 2012, reported that among approximately fifty-six thousand postmenopausal women, those with the highest dietary exposures to cadmium, were more likely to develop breast cancer than those with the lowest intake. Paradoxically, no increase in breast cancer rates was reported among obese women with higher exposure.[55]

55. Julin, Bettina, Alicja Wolk, Leif Bergkvist, Matteo Bottai, and Agneta Åkesson. "Dietary cadmium exposure and risk of postmenopausal breast cancer: a population-based prospective cohort study." *Cancer Research* 72, no. 6 (2012): 1459–1466.

CHAPTER 3

Mammography

Mammography screening is a profit-driven technology posing risks compounded by unreliability. In striking contrast, annual clinical breast examination by a trained health professional, together with monthly breast self-examination, is safe and at least as effective, and low in cost. Programs for training nurses to perform clinical breast examination (CBE), and to teach breast self-examination (BSE) are critical and well overdue.

Contrary to popular belief and assurances by the US media and the cancer establishment—the NCI and ACS—mammography is not a technique for early diagnosis. In fact, a breast cancer has usually been present for about eight years before it can be detected. Furthermore, screening should be recognized as damage control, rather than misleadingly as "secondary prevention."

The ACS has close connections to the mammography industry.[56] Five radiologists have served as ACS presidents, and in its every move, the ACS promotes the interests of the major manufacturers of mammogram machines and films, including Siemens, DuPont, General Electric, Eastman Kodak, and Piker. The mammography industry also conducts research for the ACS and its grantees, serves on advisory boards, and donates considerable funds. In virtually all its important actions, the ACS has been and remains strongly linked to the mammography industry, while ignoring or attacking the development of viable alternatives.

ACS promotion continues to lure women of all ages into mammography centers, leading them to believe that mammography is their best hope against breast cancer. A leading Massachusetts newspaper featured a photograph of two women in their twenties in an ACS advertisement that promised early detection results in a cure "nearly 100 percent of the time." An ACS communications director, questioned by journalist Kate Dempsey,

---

56. See S. S. Epstein, *The Politics of Cancer Revisited* (Fremont Center, NY: East Ridge Press, 1998).

admitted in an article published by the Massachusetts Women's Community's journal *Cancer*, "The ad isn't based on a study. When you make an advertisement, you just say what you can to get women in the door. You exaggerate a point.... Mammography today is a lucrative [and] highly competitive business."[57]

The ACS Breast Health Awareness Program sponsors television shows and other media productions touting mammography; produces advertising, promotional, and educational literature and films for hospitals, clinics, medical organizations, and doctors; and lobbies Congress for legislation promoting availability of mammography services. In virtually all of these important actions, the ACS remains strongly linked with the mammography industry, while ignoring the development of viable alternatives to mammography, particularly breast self-examination.

The ACS exposes premenopausal women to radiation hazards from mammography with little to no evidence of benefits. The ACS also fails to tell them that their breasts will change so much over time that the "baseline" images have little to no future relevance. This is truly an American Cancer Society crusade. But against whom, or rather, for whom?

MAMMOGRAM GUIDELINES, NOVEMBER 2009

1. RADIATION DOSAGE
- Chest X-ray: 1/1000 rad (1 millirad over entire chest)
- 1 mammogram: 0.2 rads (200 millirads per breast)
- 2 mammograms (routine): 0.4 rads (400 millirads per breast)
- 10 premenopausal mammograms: 4 rads (approx. 10 rads, 1 mile Hiroshima exposure)

2. NATIONAL ACADEMY OF SCIENCES, 1972

- Premenopausal breasts are highly sensitive to radiation. Each rad exposure increases breast cancer risk by 1 percent, resulting in 10 percent increased risk over ten years.

57. S. S. Epstein, "American Cancer society: The World's Wealthiest (Non-Profit) Institution," *International Journal of Health Services* 29 no. 3 (1999), 565–78.

3. CURRENT US PRACTICE: (ENDORSED BY DHHS, ACS, AND ACR; AND PAID FOR BY MEDICARE)

- Annual mammograms starting at age forty
- Against breast self-examination (BSE)

4. RECOMMENDATIONS OF THE US PREVENTIVE SERVICES TASK FORCE, 2009 (SUPPORTED BY THE NATIONAL BREAST CANCER COALITION)

- Delay mammography until age fifty
- Mammograms every two years, age fifty to seventy-five
- Against BSE at any age

5. MINIMAL ANNUAL COSTS MAMMOGRAPHY (CENSUS BUREAU ESTIMATES)

- $2.5 billion for all premenopausal women[58]
- $10 billion for all postmenopausal women
- Costs fourfold more for high-tech digital machines vs. film machines

6. MAJOR CONFLICTS OF INTEREST OF THE AMERICAN CANCER SOCIETY (ACS)

- The ACS aggressively endorsed mammography for pre- and postmenopausal women
- Evidence on ACS major conflicts of interest was made available to the *New York Times'* Gina Kolata

7. THE US VERSUS OTHER NATIONS

- No nation other than the US routinely screens premenopausal women

---

58. National Academy of Sciences– National Research Council, Advisory Committee, *Biological Effects of Ionizing Radiation (BEIR)* (Washington, DC, 1972).

8. US STATISTICS BREAST CANCER (COMMONEST CANCER IN WOMEN)

- 190,000 cases annually
- 40,000 deaths annually

NATIONAL BREAST CANCER AWARENESS MONTH

The highly publicized Breast Cancer Awareness Month (BCAM) campaign further illustrates these institutionalized conflicts of interest. Every October, ACS and NCI representatives help sponsor promotional events, hold interviews, and stress the need for mammography. The flagship of this month-long series of events is the October 15 National Mammography Day.

Conspicuously absent from the widely promoted National Breast Cancer Awareness Month is any information on environmental and other avoidable causes of breast cancer. This is no accident. Zeneca Pharmaceuticals—a spin-off of Imperial Chemical Industries—is one of the world's largest manufacturers of chlorinated and other industrial chemicals, including those incriminated as causes of breast cancer. Zeneca has also been the sole multimillion-dollar funder of the National Breast Cancer Awareness Month since its inception in 1984, besides the sole manufacturer of tamoxifen, the world's top-selling anticancer and breast cancer "prevention" drug, with $400 million in annual sales. Furthermore, Zeneca recently assumed direct management of eleven cancer centers in US hospitals, and Zeneca owns a 50 percent stake in these centers, known collectively as Salick Health Care.

The link between the ACS, NCI, and Zeneca is especially strong when it comes to tamoxifen. The ACS and NCI continue to aggressively promote tamoxifen, which is the cornerstone of its minimal prevention program. On March 7, 1997, the NCI Press Office released a four-page statement "For Response to Inquiries on Breast Cancer." The brief section on prevention reads:

> Researchers are looking for a way to prevent breast cancer in women at high risk . . . A large study [is underway] to see if the drug Tamoxifen will reduce cancer risk in women age 60 or

older and in women 35 to 59 who have a pattern of risk factors for breast cancer. This study is also a model for future studies of cancer prevention. Studies of diet and nutrition could also lead to preventive strategies.[59]

Since Zeneca influences every leaflet, poster, publication, and commercial of the National Breast Cancer Awareness Month, it is no wonder that such information and publications, made no mention of carcinogenic industrial chemicals and their relation to breast cancer. Imperial Chemical Industries, Zeneca's parent company, profits by manufacturing breast cancer-causing chemicals. Zeneca profits from treatment of breast cancer, and hopes to profit still more from the prospects of large-scale national use of tamoxifen for breast cancer prevention. National Breast Cancer Awareness Month is a masterful public relations coup for Zeneca, providing the company with unmerited goodwill, besides money from millions of women.

US PREVENTATIVE SERVICES TASK FORCE (USPSTF): RECOMMENDED SCREENING FOR BREAST CANCER, DECEMBER 2009

SUMMARY OF RECOMMENDATION AND EVIDENCE

- The USPSTF recommends biennial screening mammography for women aged fifty to seventy-four years. (Grade: B recommendation.)
- The decision to start regular, biennial screening mammography before the age of fifty years should be an individual one and take patient context into account, including the patient's values regarding specific benefits and harms. (Grade: C recommendation.)
- The USPSTF concludes that the current evidence is insufficient to assess the additional benefits and harms of screening mammography in women seventy-five years or older. (Grade: I Statement.)
- The USPSTF warns against teaching BSE. (Grade: D recommendation.)

59. S. S. Epstein, "World's Wealthiest Nonprofit Institution," *International Journal of Health Services* 29 no. 3 (1999).

- The USPSTF concludes that the current evidence is insufficient to assess the additional benefits and harms of clinical breast examination (CBE) beyond screening mammography in women forty years or older. (Grade: I Statement.)
- The USPSTF concludes that the current evidence is insufficient to assess the additional benefits and harms of either digital mammography or magnetic resonance imaging (MRI) instead of film mammography as screening modalities for breast cancer. (Grade: I Statement.)

BREAST EXAMS ARE JUST AS EFFECTIVE AND SAFER THAN MAMMOGRAPHY SCREENING

Contrary to extensive media coverage, a Chinese trial on monthly BSE does not disprove its effectiveness in preventing breast cancer deaths. Furthermore, the study is irrelevant to the well-documented effectiveness of BSE, especially when combined with annual CBE by a trained professional.

Contrary to media reports that the Chinese self-exams were done regularly, the researchers admit that BSE was practiced "roughly every 4–5 months" during the first four to five years of the ten-year trial, and with unknown frequency subsequently. The researchers also admitted evidence, from numerous studies over the last two decades, that: breast cancers detected by BSE "tend to be diagnosed at an earlier stage and to be smaller than cancers diagnosed in the absence of any screening"; that women "practicing BSE tend to have their tumors diagnosed at an earlier stage than women who do not report practicing BSE"; that "women who regularly and competently practice BSE are more likely to find their tumors themselves than women who practice BSE less diligently"; and that tumor size is "inversely associated with the frequency of practicing BSE."[60]

Surprisingly, in their listing of forty-four references, the researchers omit reference to the landmark 2000 Canadian National Breast Cancer Screening Study that demonstrates the effectiveness of breast exams in reducing breast cancer mortality. This evidence is confirmed in an editorial commenting on the Chinese study publication: "There is evidence that excellent physical

60. David B. Thomas et al., "Randomized trial of breast self-examination in Shanghai," *Journal of the National Cancer Institute* 94 no. 19 (2002), 1445–57.

examination practice, whether BSE or CBE, may indeed be effective. Not only is there case-control evidence that competent BSE may reduce mortality, there is also randomized, controlled trial evidence that CBE done by trained nurse-examiners may be as effective as mammography in reducing breast cancer mortality. The addition of annual mammography screening to physical examination has no impact on breast cancer mortality."[61]

Over the ten-year period of the Chinese trial, the incidence of benign tumors was approximately twice as high in the BSE group than in the controls. This contrasts with a threefold higher incidence noted in the Canadian mammography group. Such false positives, or overdiagnosis, usually leads to unnecessary biopsies and even surgery.

The routine practice of taking two films of each breast annually over ten years, results in approximately 0.5 rad (radiation absorbed dose) exposure per year. This is about five hundred times greater than exposure from a single chest X-ray, broadly focused on the entire chest rather than narrowly on the breast. Moreover, the premenopausal breast is highly sensitive to radiation. Each rad exposure increases risks of breast cancer by about 1 percent, with a cumulative 5 percent increased risk for each breast over a decade's screening. So, a premenopausal woman having annual mammograms over ten years is exposed to roughly 5 rads. This is the approximate level of radiation received by a Japanese woman a mile or so away from where the Hiroshima or Nagasaki atom bombs were detonated.

Radiation risks are increased by fourfold for the 1 to 2 percent of women who may be unknowing and silent carriers of the A-T (ataxia-telangiectasia) gene,[62] and thus highly sensitive to the carcinogenic effects of radiation. By some estimates, this accounts for up to 20 percent of all breast cancers diagnosed annually.

Of additional concern, missed cancers are common in premenopausal women due to the density of their breasts. Mammography also entails tight and often painful breast compression, particularly in premenopausal women. This may lead to the rupture of small blood vessels in or around small undetected breast cancers, and the lethal distant spread of malignant cells.

61. Russell Harris and Linda S. Kinsinger, "Routinely Teaching BSE Is Dead. What Does This Mean?" *Journal of the National Cancer Institute* 94 no. 19 (2002), 1420-1.

62. M. Swift, D. Morrell, E. Cromartie, et al., "The incidence and gene frequency of ataxia-telangiectasia in the United States," *Am J Hum Genet* 39 (1986): 573-83.

As early as 1985, the ACS admitted that most breast cancers are first recognized by the women themselves. "At least 90 percent of women who develop breast cancer discover the tumors themselves."[63]

Furthermore, an analysis of several 1993 studies showed that women who regularly performed monthly BSEs detected their cancers much earlier than those who failed to do so. However, the ACS and radiologists still claim that "no studies have clearly shown a benefit of using BSE."[64]

Finally, and not surprisingly, premenopausal mammography is practiced by no nation other than the United States. As reported by the British journalist Liz Savage, in 2009 "*The Times of London* published a letter reprimanding the UK's National Health Service (NHS) for not providing women with adequate information about the risks of screening mammography. Signed by nearly two dozen physicians, researchers, and patient advocates, the letter described 'the harms associated with early detection of breast cancer by screening that are not widely acknowledged.' The most important of these harms are over-diagnosis . . . and its frequent consequence, over-treatment."[65]

THE FDA BELATEDLY ADMITS RADIATION RISKS, BUT NOT DANGERS OF MAMMOGRAPHY

On February 9, 2010, the Food and Drug Administration (FDA) announced that it would take stringent action to regulate "the most potent forms of medical radiation,"[66] particularly those from an increasingly popular new scanning device, known as the cone-beam CT scanner. The FDA also warned that such radiation is unsafe and equivalent to that about of four hundred chest X-rays, 0.4 rads (radiation absorbed dose), and "can increase a person's lifetime cancer risk." Information on this risk is not new. It dates back to the late Dr. John Gofman's explicit warning in his 1999 monograph, "Radiation From Medical Procedures and the Pathogenesis of Cancer."

63. Walter Ross, *Crusade: The Official History of the American Cancer Society* (Westminster, MD: Arbor House, 1987) 96.

64. Andrea Walker Gehrke, "Brest Self-Examination: A Mixed Message." *Journal of the National Cancer Institute* 92 no. 14 (2000): 1120–1.

65. Liz Savage, "Invitation or Summons? UK Debate Surrounds Messages About Mammography." *Journal of the National Cancer Institute* 101 no. 13 (2009): 912–3.

66. Walt Bogdanich, "FDA to Increase Oversight of Medical Radiation," *The New York Times*, February 9, 2010.

However, the FDA still remains strangely unaware that radiation from routine premenopausal mammography poses significant and cumulative risks of breast cancer. This is also contrary to its conventional assurances that radiation exposure from mammography is trivial, about 1/1,000 of a rad, and similar to just that from a chest X-ray. However, the routine practice of taking two films of each breast results in exposure of about 0.4 rads, focused on the breast rather than on the entire chest. Thus, premenopausal women undergoing annual screening over a ten-year period are exposed to a total of at least 4 rads for each breast, at least eight times greater radiation than the FDA's "cancer risk" level.

This alarming information is not new. In 1972, the prestigious National Academy of Sciences warned that the overall risks of breast cancer increase by one percent for every single rad exposure. This totals a 10 percent risk from ten years annual premenopausal mammography. These warnings were emphasized in my 1978 *The Politics of Cancer*, "Whatever you may be told, refuse routine mammograms, especially if you are pre-menopausal. The X-rays may increase your chances of getting cancer."

A 1993 Swedish study involving forty-two thousand women showed that those under the age of fifty-five who received regular premenopausal mammography experienced a 29 percent greater risk of dying from breast cancer. Based on a detailed review of these and a wide range of other such studies, the late Dr. John Gofman published an analysis in his classic 1995 book, *Preventing Breast Cancer*. He stressed that medical radiation is probably the single most important cause of the modern breast cancer epidemic.

These warnings were further detailed in a 2001 article, with some fifty scientific references, "The Dangers and Unreliability of Mammography: Breast Self Examination As A Safe Effective and Practical Alternative,"[67] published in the prestigious *International Journal of Health Services*. This was co-authored by Dr. Rosalie Bertell, a leading international expert on the dangers of radiation, the late Barbara Seaman, founder and leader of the women's breast cancer movement, and myself. An analysis of several 1993 studies showed that women who regularly performed monthly BSEs,

67. S. S. Epstein, R. Bertell, and B. Seaman, "The Dangers and Unreliability of Mammography," *International Journal of Health Science* 31 no. 3 (2001): 605–15.

particularly following training by qualified nurses, detected their cancers much earlier than those who failed to do so.

This wide range of concerns on the still unrecognized dangers of routine premenopausal mammography are critical, especially in view of the current high incidence of breast cancer. Disturbingly, this has increased by about 20 percent since 1975 in spite of routine premenopausal mammography, and its multi-billion dollar insurance costs. Such funds should instead be directed to establishing BSE training clinics nationwide. Not surprisingly, the prestigious *Chronicle of Philanthropy*, the nation's leading charity watch dog, has warned the obvious. The ACS "is more interested in accumulating wealth than saving lives."

DANGERS OF MAMMOGRAPHY

Mammography poses a wide range of risks of which women still remain uninformed.

RADIATION RISKS

Radiation from routine premenopausal mammography poses significant cumulative risks of initiating and promoting breast cancer. As emphasized over three decades ago, the premenopausal breast is highly sensitive to radiation, each rad exposure increasing breast cancer risk by 1 percent. This results in a cumulative 10 percent increased risk over ten years of premenopausal screening, usually from ages forty to fifty. Risks are even greater for "baseline" screening at younger ages, for which there is no evidence of any future relevance. Furthermore, breast cancer risks from mammography are up to fourfold higher for the 1 to 2 percent of women who are silent carriers of the A-T (ataxia-telangiectasia) gene, and thus highly sensitive to the carcinogenic effects of radiation. This accounts for up to 20 percent of all breast cancers diagnosed annually in the United States.

Delays in Diagnostic Mammography
As increasing numbers of premenopausal women are responding to the ACS's aggressively promoted screening, imaging centers are becoming

flooded and overwhelmed. As a result, patients referred for diagnostic mammography are now experiencing potentially dangerous delays, up to several months, before they can be examined.

UNRELIABILITY OF MAMMOGRAPHY

Falsely Negative Mammograms

Missed cancers are particularly common in premenopausal women owing to the dense and highly glandular structure of their breasts, and increased proliferation late in their menstrual cycle. Missed cancers are also common in postmenopausal women on estrogen replacement therapy (ERT), as about 20 percent develop breast densities that make their mammograms as difficult to read as those of premenopausal women.

Interval Cancers

About one-third of all cancers, and more still of premenopausal cancers are aggressive, even to the extent of doubling in size in one month. These cancers are more likely to metastasize in the interval between successive annual mammograms. Premenopausal women particularly can thus be lulled into a false sense of security by a supposedly negative result on an annual mammogram and fail to seek medical advice.

Falsely Positive Mammogram

Mistakenly diagnosed cancers are particularly common in premenopausal women, and also in postmenopausal women on ERT, resulting in needless anxiety, more mammograms, and unnecessary biopsies. For childless women with multiple high-risk factors including a strong family history, prolonged use of the contraceptive pill, and early menarche—just those groups that are most strongly urged to have annual mammograms—the cumulative risk of false positives increases to "as high as 100 percent" over a decade's screening.

Overdiagnosis

Overdiagnosis and subsequent overtreatment are among the major risks of mammography. The widespread and virtually unchallenged acceptance of screening has resulted in a dramatic increase in the diagnosis of a preinvasive cancer, ductal carcinoma-in-situ (DCIS), with a current estimated incidence of about forty thousand annually. DCIS is usually recognized pin point calcifications and generally treated by lumpectomy and radiation or even mastectomy and chemotherapy. However, some 80 percent of all DCIS cases never become invasive even if left untreated. Furthermore, the breast cancer mortality from DCIS is the same, just about 1 percent for women diagnosed and treated early as for those diagnosed later following the development of invasive cancer.

FAILURE TO REDUCE BREAST CANCER MORTALITY

The long-standing claims that routine mammography screening allows early detection and treatment of breast cancer, thereby reducing mortality, are, at best, highly questionable. In fact, the overwhelming majority of breast cancers are unaffected by early detection, either because they are aggressive or slow growing. There is also supportive evidence that the major variable predicting survival is "biological determinism—a combination of virulence of an individual tumor together with the host's immune response," rather than just early detection.[68]

Claims for the benefit of screening mammography in reducing breast cancer mortality have been based on eight international controlled trials involving about five hundred thousand women. However, specialized or meta-analysis of these trials revealed that only two, based on sixty-six thousand postmenopausal women, were adequately randomized to allow statistically valid conclusions. Based on these trials, it was concluded that "there is no reliable evidence that screening decreases breast cancer mortality—not even a tendency towards an effect."[69] Accordingly, the authors concluded that there is no longer any justification for screening mammography. Further evidence was detailed at the May 6, 2001, annual meeting of the National Breast Cancer Coalition in Washington, DC, and published in the July 2001 report of the Nordic Cochrane Centre.

---

68. B. H. Lerner, "Public health then and now: Great expectations: Historical perspectives on genetic brest cancer testing." *American Journal of Public Health* 89 no. 6 (1999): 938–44.

69. P. C. Gotzsche and O. Olsen, "Is screening for breast cancer with mammography justifiable?" *Lancet* 355 no. 9198 (2000): 129–34.

THE UNITED STATES VERSUS OTHER NATIONS

No nation other than the United States routinely screens premenopausal women by mammography. In this context, it should be noted that the January 1997 National Institutes of Health Consensus Conference did not recommend premenopausal screening, a decision that the NCI, but not the ACS, accepted. However, under pressure from Congress, the NCI reversed its decision some three months later in favor of premenopausal screening.

The US overkill extends to the standard practice of taking two or more mammograms per breast annually in postmenopausal women. This contrasts with the more restrained European practice of a single view every two to three years.

COSTS OF SCREENING

If all US premenopausal women, about twenty million according to the Census Bureau, submitted to annual mammograms, annual costs would be over $2.5 billion. These costs would be increased to $10 billion, about 5 percent of the $200 billion 2001 Medicare budget, if all postmenopausal women were also screened annually. Such costs will further increase some fourfold if the industry, enthusiastically supported by radiologists, succeeds in efforts to replace film machines, costing about $100,000, with the latest high-tech digital machines. Those were approved by the FDA in November 2000 and now cost over $400,000. Digital mammography thus poses major threats to the financially strained Medicare system. Inflationary costs aside, there is no evidence of the greater effectiveness of digital than film mammography

The comparative cost of CBE and mammography in the 1992 Canadian Breast Cancer Screening Study was reported to be 1 to 3.[70] However, this ratio ignores the high costs of capital items including buildings, equipment, and mobile vans, let alone the much greater hidden costs of unnecessary biopsies, specialized staff training, and programs for quality control and professional accreditation. This ratio could be even more favorable for

70. A. B. Miller, C. J. Baines, T. To, and C. Wall, "Canadian National Breast Cancer Screening Study," *Canadian Medical Association Journal* 147 no. 10 (1992): 1459–88.

CBE and BSE instruction if both were conducted by trained nurses. The excessive costs of mammography screening should be diverted away from industry to breast cancer prevention and other women's health programs.

NEEDED REFORMS

Mammography is a striking paradigm of the capture of unsuspecting women by run-away powerful technological and pharmaceutical global industries, with the complicity of ACS, and the rollover mainstream media. Promotion of the multibillion-dollar mammography screening industry has also become a diversionary flag around which legislators and women's product corporations can rally, protesting how much they care about women, while studiously avoiding any reference to avoidable risks of breast cancer.

Screening mammography should be phased out in favor of annual CBE and monthly BSE, as they are effective, safe, and low-cost alternatives, while diagnostic mammography should be available when so indicated. Such action is all the more critical and overdue in view of the still poorly recognized evidence that screening mammography fails to decrease breast cancer mortality.

Networks of CBE and BSE clinics, staffed by trained nurses, should be established nationally. These low-cost clinics would further empower women by providing them with scientific evidence on breast cancer risks and prevention. This information is of critical importance in view of the continued high incidence of breast cancers. The multibillion-dollar US insurance and Medicare costs of mammography should be diverted to outreach and research on breast cancer prevention, along with other women's health programs.

SELECTIVE JUSTIFICATION FOR PREMENOPAUSAL MAMMOGRAPHY

As reported in the May 4, 2012 issue of *The Cancer Letter*, based on a review of over sixty publications by the Breast Cancer Surveillance Consortium, routine premenopausal screening mammography may be justified for premenopausal women at significantly increased risk of breast cancer.

These include women with a first-degree relative with breast cancer, more than one first degree relatives with breast cancer, or a first-degree relative diagnosed before the age of fifty.

Apart from ignoring the role of avoidable carcinogenic dietary contaminants, the NCI and ACS have also failed to investigate the carcinogenic hazards of mammography, particularly the relation between increasing breast cancer rates and the high-dose mammograms administered without warning to some three hundred thousand women in the 1970s Breast Cancer Detection and Demonstration Program (BCDDP). A confidential memo by a senior NCI physician in charge of the screening program may explain why, despite warnings by the National Academy of Sciences in 1972 and by the NCI's own key scientific staff, women were not warned of this risk. The memo may also account for the cancer establishment's enthusiasm for the BCDDP program: "Both the [ACS] and NCI will gain a great deal of favorable publicity because they are bringing research findings to the public and applying them. This will assist in obtaining more research funds for basic research and clinical research which is sorely needed."[71]

It may be further noted that the NCI has also failed to adequately explore safe alternatives to mammography, particularly transillumination with infrared light scanning. This is all the more serious in view of recent reports of excess breast cancer mortality in premenopausal women following mammography, together with accumulating evidence of its diagnostic ineffectiveness in younger women, including the recent large-scale Canadian study by Cornelia Baines and Anthony Miller: "There is no evidence to support introduction of service mammography for women under 50, and some may argue that there should be a moratorium on all mammography for symptom-free women in this age group outside randomized control trials."[72]

The NCI still ignores carcinogenic dietary contaminants and high-dose mammography in the 1970s as preventable causes of breast cancer. Meanwhile, the NCI designates its tamoxifen chemoprevention trail as "primary

---

71. From "Minutes of BCDDP Special Meeting for Discussion of Project Protocol," January 9 1974. Given to John C Bailar III following a Freedom of Information request. Cited in Robert Aronowitz's *Unnatural History* (Cambridge University Press, 2007).

72. C. Baines, A. Miller, et al., "Canadian National Breast Cancer Screening Study: First screen results as predictors of future breast cancer risk," *Cancer Epidemiology, Biomarkers, and Prevention* 2 no. 1 (1993): 1–19.

cancer prevention."[73] In May 1992, the NCI initiated this trial on sixteen thousand healthy women at increased risk of breast cancer due to familial and more questionable reasons, including being over the age of sixty. The tamoxifen trial is a prospective experiment in human carcinogenesis whose scientific invalidity is compounded by a misleading patient consent form, trivializing risks and exaggerating benefits; participating oncologists and institutions clearly risk future malpractice claims.

Tamoxifen, which is structurally related to DES, induces covalent DNA adducts in rodents, thus making "this drug a poor choice for the chronic preventive treatment of breast cancer."[74] Tamoxifen induced 15 percent of liver tumors in rats at doses equivalent to the daily 20 mg low dose in human adjuvant therapy, and 71 percent at the higher 40 mg dose; these tumors were highly malignant. This experimental evidence of potent carcinogenicity is confirmed by two case reports of liver cancer among ninety-three women receiving 40 mg tamoxifen doses in the Stockholm adjuvant therapy trials, and more strikingly by several reports of endometrial cancer, particularly in the Stockholm trial documenting a 6.4 relative risk of endometrial cancer. It should further be emphasized that the median follow-up for all the seven reported tamoxifen trials was only eighty months; very few healthy women have taken the drug for more than five years. Thus, tamoxifen may well be a much more potent human carcinogen than is currently recognized.

73. B Fisher et al., "Tamoxifen for prevention of breast cancer," *Journal of the National Cancer Institute* 90 no. 18 (1998): 1371–88.

74. X. Han, J. G. Liehr, "Induction of Covalent DNA Adducts in Rodents by Tamoxifen," *Cancer Research* 52 no. 5 (1992): 1360–3.

Note: certain parcels of information of a statistical nature are repeated in some of the articles reprinted below. Since I wanted to include these articles here exactly as they originally appeared, such occasional repetition is unavoidable and, I hope, harmless.

CHAPTER 4

Newspaper Articles 1992–2002

June 22, 1992	Perspective on Medicine: A Travesty, at Women's Expense (*LA Times*)
December 28, 1993	Radiation's Risks (*NY Times*)
March 20, 1994	A Needless New Risk of Breast Cancer (*LA Times*)
September 9,1994	Women At Risk Are Still in the Dark (*LA Times*)
October 26, 1997	Awareness Month Keeps Women Perilously Unaware (*Chicago Tribune*)
April 19, 1998	Failure to Fully Document Risks of Osteoporosis Drug is "Reckless"(*Chicago*
June 5, 1998	No Safety in These Implant Numbers (*Chicago Tribune*)
March 14, 2001	Mammography's Mixed Blessings (*Chicago Tribune*)
February 5, 2002	Mammography Doesn't Come Without Risk (*LA Times*)

March 28, 1992, *Los Angeles Times*
MAMMOGRAPHY RADIATES DOUBT[75]

It has been widely (and with reason) charged that the makers and marketers of silicone breast implants, and self-interested plastic surgeons, made women their guinea pigs. But what of that other, and greater, scourge of women, breast cancer? There is reason to believe that, women are equally ill-served by the cancer establishment, especially in its unrelenting promotion of mammography.

Breast cancer now strikes one in nine women, a dramatic increase from the one in 20 measured in 1950. This year, 180,000 new cases and 46,000 deaths are expected. Hearings scheduled Feb. 5 in Washington by

---

75. Republished in the *International Journal of Health Services*, Volume 22, 1992.

the Breast Cancer Coalition, an advocacy group loosely modeled on AIDS activists, could not seem more timely.

The coalition wants more federal funding for the National Cancer Institute (NCI) to increase its research into the causes and treatment of breast cancer, and to improve delivery of breast health care—including diagnostic screening. In pursuing these goals, the coalition has been co-opted into supporting the policies of the cancer Establishment—NCI and the American Cancer Society—which is fixated on basic research, diagnosis and treatment. Cancer prevention receives only an estimated 5% of the annual $1.8 billion NCI budget.

Breast cancer is not the only cancer on the rise. While its incidence has increased 57% since 1950, overall cancer has increased 44%, now striking one in three people and killing one in four. Male colon cancer is up 60%, testis, prostate and kidney cancer up 100%, and other cancers, such as malignant melanoma and multiple myeloma, more than 100%. The cancer Establishment trivializes evidence linking these increasing rates with avoidable exposure to cancer-causing industrial chemicals and radiation that permeate our environment—food, water, air and workplace.

The cancer Establishment maintains, on tenuous evidence, that a fatty diet itself is a major cause of breast cancer, while ignoring contaminants in fat. Carcinogenic pesticides, such as the highly persistent chlordane and dieldrin, which concentrate in animals fats, are known to cause breast cancer in rodents. Elevated levels of DDT and PCBs are found in human breast cancer deaths in younger women recently dropped by 30%, despite a substantial increase in consumption of animal fat. This drop followed, and seems linked to, regulations that reduced previously high levels of DDT and related pesticides in dairy products. These pesticides act by mimicking the action of estrogens or by increasing estrogen production in the body, which in turn increases the risk of breast cancer. A related concern is lifelong exposure of all women to estrogenic contaminants in animal fat; because of their unregulated use as growth-promoting additives in cattle feed.

In 1977, NCI's director of endocrinology, Dr. Roy Hertz, warned, without effect, of breast cancer risks from these contaminants.

More ominous is the enthusiastic endorsement by the cancer Establishment of massive nationwide expansion of X-ray mammography, including routine annual screening. While there is a general consensus that mammography improves early cancer detection and survival in post-menopausal women, no such benefit is demonstrable for younger women.

Furthermore, there is clear evidence that the breast, particularly in pre-menopausal women, is highly sensitive to radiation, with estimates of increased risk of breast cancer of up to 1% for every rad (radiation absorbed dose) unit of X-ray exposure. This project up to a 20% increased cancer risk for a woman who, in the 1970s, received 10 annual mammograms of an average two rads each. In spite of this, up to 40% of women over 40 have had mammograms since the mid-1960s, some annually and some with exposures of 5 to 10 rads in a single screening from older, high-dose equipment.

Significant studies on radiation risks to the breast have been well known since the late 1960s, including evidence that mammography, especially in younger women, was likely to cause more cancers than could be detected. A confidential memo by Dr. Nathaniel Berlin, a senior NCI physician in charge of large scale mammography screening, in 1973 may explain why women were not warned of this risk: "Both the [American Cancer Society] and NCI will gain a great deal of favorable publicity [from screening, and] . . . this will assist in obtaining more research funds for basic and clinical research which is sorely needed."

Thus, once again, suspect technology was applied to women on a large scale, in spite of clear warning signals and with insufficient knowledge of the likely consequences. (On a smaller scale, but even more ethically appalling, was the use until last April of industrial polyurethane foam to coat silicone breast inserts, despite clear evidence that its manufacturing contaminants and break-down products were carcinogenic. As with mammography, no serious studies have been launched to find out what happened to women in whom the foam was implanted, or indeed to women carrying any type of silicone implant.)

The risks of mammography, especially for premenopausal women, per-sist with the lower radiation doses (about one-half rad per screening) found in modern facilities with dedicated equipment and licensed operators. A large Canadian study conducted from 1980 to 1988 found a 52% increase in early breast cancer deaths in women aged 40 to 50 who had 10 annual mammograms, compared to women given just physical examinations. More recent concern comes from evidence that 1% of women carry a gene that increases their breast cancer risk from radiation four-fold.

The coalition should insist that the NCI and American Cancer Society initiate an immediate, large-scale, well-publicized study to further investigate the role of past mammography in increasing breast cancer rates, and to investigate future cancer risk from mammography as currently conducted under widely varying conditions. Women should also be informed of their X-ray exposure and individual and cumulative risks each time they undergo mammography. The coalition should demand an immediate ban on obsolete high-dose X-ray equipment, and the abandonment of routine mammograms on premenopausal women.

The coalition should also encourage a crash program to develop and make available safe alternatives to mammography, apart from physical examination. Two that show the most promise are magnetic resonance imaging and trans-illumination with infrared light. The expansion of mammography should be put on hold, especially in view of the 1991 conclusion of the General Accounting Office that there are more than enough machines to meet the screening needs of American women.

The Breast Cancer Coalition represents a welcome trend toward active grass-roots involvement in public health. However, its current goals are too narrowly defined within the context of existing perspectives and institutional policies. The coalition needs broader and more radical strategies if it is to reverse the modern epidemic of breast cancer.

June 22, 1992, *Los Angeles Times*
PERSPECTIVES ON MEDICINE: A TRAVESTY, AT WOMEN'S EXPENSE

The government's National Cancer Institute this spring launched a large-scale breast-cancer prevention trial, recruiting thousands of healthy women at increased risk of breast cancer—including those with close relatives with the disease, and also anyone over 60. Half are to be treated with tamoxifen, a potent chemotherapy drug; the remainder will get a placebo. The NCI believes tamoxifen can reduce breast cancers by 30%, while also reducing heart attacks and preventing osteoporosis.

With one in nine women expected to develop breast cancer over a lifetime, the trial would seem worthy of unqualified support. However, the evidence that tamoxifen can prevent breast cancer is largely wishful thinking. To make matters worse, the risks to healthy women of a wide range of serious complications, including uterine cancer, fatal liver cancer, liver failure, life-threatening blood clots and crippling menopausal symptoms are unacceptable. This trial must be halted in its tracks.

The NCI's rationale is that tamoxifen, which is modestly successful in treating breast cancer, appears to reduce the risk of new cancers of the other breast. This benefit has only been seen in some patients in about half of the studies that have been done. The protection also appears largely restricted to post-menopausal women. However, the NCI ignores this and misleadingly offers healthy younger women the hope of prevention.

In addition, Swedish studies suggest that tamoxifen *increases* mortality in post-menopausal women who do develop cancer in the other breast during treatment; these cancers were highly aggressive and treatment-resistant. This evidence appears confirmed by studies showing that while tamoxifen reduces breast cancer in rats, cancers that do develop are highly malignant. There are also questions concerning whether heart benefits actually exist, and to what extent.

If tamoxifen's effectiveness were the only question, our alarm would not be so great. But the drug is implicated in a range of serious and sometimes life-threatening complications, although the NCI dismisses these as "infrequently severe."

Tamoxifen triples the risk of uterine cancer, even in patients followed for relatively short periods. Reaching a new low in medical sexism, statistician Richard Peto, a leading British supporter of the trial, dismisses the risk as "no big deal," since uterine cancer is curable by hysterectomy.

Tamoxifen is also a "rip-roaring liver carcinogen," according to Gary Williams, medical director of the American Health Foundation, inducing aggressive cancers in 100% of rats at high doses and 20% at lower doses equivalent to those being used in the prevention trial. This is acknowledged by the drug's manufacturer, ICI Americas, Inc. The prestigious British Medical Research Council warns of the absence of any safety margin at the trial dose. Yet the NCI misleadingly trivializes evidence of liver cancer in rats and ignores reports of two liver cancers in women at just double the dose used in the trials. Tamoxifen also promotes liver cancer in rats previously exposed to low doses of other carcinogens.

Moreover, as the British council emphasized, "Few women have received tamoxifen for longer than five to seven years, whereas the maximum incidence of liver tumors induced by known carcinogens occurs at eight to 10 years." Indeed, it is probable that a significant number of healthy women receiving tamoxifen may die from liver cancer after a decade or so.

Recent Swedish data suggest a more than 50% increase in new cancers, including gastrointestinal, among breast cancer patients treated with tamoxifen.

Shortly before the NCI started its trial, the blue-ribbon British Committee on Safety of Medicines reported five cases of liver failure with four fatalities, five hepatitis with one fatality and 11 other liver complications in breast-cancer patients treated with tamoxifen. Previously undisclosed similar evidence has just been obtained from the US Food and Drug Administration.

The NCI recognizes a sixfold risk of often-fatal blood-clotting problems with tamoxifen, but the trial's coordinator suggests, with no supporting evidence, that this is due not to tamoxifen itself, but to "the interactive effect of (other) chemotherapy." Sometimes-severe menopausal symptoms, including hot flashes and vaginal discharge, are other recognized complications that the NCI seeks to downplay.

December 28, 1993, *New York Times*
RADIATION'S RISKS

To the Editor:

The debate on mammography reflects flawed science and misplaced emotionalism (front page, Dec. 27). Despite more than three decades of large-scale experience in the United States and elsewhere, no study has shown any benefit for mammography in premenopausal, as opposed to postmenopausal women.

But substantial documentation on radiation risks to the breast has accumulated since the late 1980's. This includes evidence that mammography, especially in younger women whose breasts are sensitive to radiation, is likely to cause more cancer than could be detected. These risks are greater in women who unknowingly carry the A-T gene, which substantially increases risks from radiation cancer.

There is also evidence that radiation can synergize the carcinogenic effects of estrogens from sources such as oral contraceptives.

As an editorial in The Lancet, the British medical journal, emphasizes, recent studies have shown excess breast cancer mortality in premenopausal women receiving repeated mammography. Rather than pressuring the Clinton Administration for ineffective and hazardous mammography in younger women, the American Cancer Society and its supporters would do well to encourage a program to develop and use safer alternatives, such as transillumination with infrared light scanning and magnetic resonance imaging, besides emphasis on training in regular breast self-examination. Meanwhile, there is no reason to extend insurance coverage for premenopausal mammography.

March 20, 1994, *Los Angeles Times*

A NEEDLESS NEW RISK OF BREAST CANCER

The Food and Drug Administration recently warned dairy producers, distributors and retailers against "hormone-free" labels on milk from cows that have not been given the biotech milk-production stimulant known as recombinant bovine growth hormone. The FDA states that such labeling could be "false or misleading" under federal law, as there is "no significant difference between milk from treated and untreated cows." Monsanto, maker of the hormone, is already suing one large Midwest milk producer for using the label.

The confusing FDA guidelines were, according to the consumer publication Daily Citizen, written by Deputy Commissioner Michael Taylor, a former counsel for Monsanto and a biotech umbrella organization. The guidelines are scientifically flawed and reckless and reflect flagrant disregard of consumers' right to know. Furthermore, the FDA ignores evidence linking milk from treated cows with increased risk of breast cancer. The concerns, based on published research:

- The biotech hormone induces a marked and sustained increase in levels of insulin-like growth factor-1, or IGF-1, in cow's milk.
- IGF-1 regulates cell growth, division and differentiation, particularly in infants. While human and normal bovine IGF-1 are identical, they are largely bound to protein and thus probably less biologically active than

the unbound IGF-1 in treated milk.

- IGF-1 is not destroyed by pasteurization or digestion and is readily absorbed across the intestinal wall. In a 1990 FDA publication disclosing toxicity tests conducted by Monsanto, feeding the hormone (trade name Posilac) to mature rats for only two weeks resulted in statistically significant increases in body and liver weights and bone length. These effects were seen at a small fraction of injected doses given to control rats. But by gerrymandering these explicit data, the FDA alleged that IGF-1 "lacks oral toxicity."
- Neither the FDA nor Monsanto has investigated the effects of long-term feeding of IGF-1 and treated milk on growth, or on more sensitive sub-cellular effects in infant rats or infants of any other species.

Cows injected with the biotech hormone show heavy localization of IGF-1 in breast (udder) epithelial cells; this does not occur in untreated cows.

- IGF-1 induces rapid division and multiplication of normal human breast epithelial cells in tissue cultures.
- It is highly likely that IGF-1 promotes transformation of normal breast epithelium to breast cancer.
- IGF-1 maintains the malignancy of human breast-cancer cells, including their invasiveness and ability to spread to distant organs.
- The breast tissues of female fetuses and infants are sensitive to hormonal influences. Imprinting by IGF-1 may increase future breast-cancer risks and sensitivity of the breast to subsequent unrelated risks such as mammography and the carcinogenic and estrogen-like effects of pesticide residues in food, particularly in premenopausal women.

These concerns are not new. In a 1989 letter to the FDA, I warned that the effects of IGF-1 "could include premature growth stimulation in infants, [breast enlargement] in young children and breast cancer in adult females." More recently, the Council on Scientific Affairs of the American Medical Association stated: "Further studies will be required to determine whether the ingestion of higher-than-normal concentrations of bovine insulin-like growth factor is safe for children, adolescents, and adults." The opposite of "further study" is uncontrolled, unlabeled sales of treated milk to unwitting consumers.

Apart from risks of breast cancer and other IGF-1 effects, the FDA and industry have down-played additional differences between hormonal and non-hormonal milk. The FDA- approved label insert for Posilac, a pamphlet that only dairy farmers see, admits that its "use is associated with increased frequency of use of medication in cows for mastitis and other health problems." Monsanto's own data further show up to an 80% incidence of mastitis, an udder infection, in hormone-treated cattle and resulting contamination of milk with statistically significant levels of pus; this will necessitate virtually routine use of antibiotics, with attendant risks of allergic reactions and antibiotic resistance.

Congress should insist that, at the very least, the FDA immediately revoke its restrictions on labeling of milk from untreated cows. More prudently, it should ban the use of these hormones.

September 9, 1994, *Los Angeles Times*
WOMEN AT RISK ARE STILL IN THE DARK

Last week's establishment of a $4.25-billion settlement fund seems to add finality to the breast-implant controversy, even though the judge in the case believes that the amount, contributed by manufacturers, will be insufficient for current claims. The settlement also is insufficient because it ignores the risk of breast cancers developing decades later.

The Food and Drug Administration has consistently downplayed any cancer risk from silicone gel implants. But the agency's sanguine position is contradicted by substantial research, including its own. Why is no one sounding an alarm? Why is no one informing women of their risk and offering all women with breast implants the option of removal?

Studies by manufacturer Dow Corning, discovered in 1987 FDA inspections, and showed that silicone-gel injection induced malignant tumors in rats. Internal memoranda by FDA scientists concluded that "while there is no direct proof that silicone causes cancer in humans, there is considerable reason to suspect that it can do so" and urged that "a medical alert be issued to warn the public of the possibility of malignancy following long-term implant(ation)." The FDA's response was to reassign the report's writers.

Another report, in the July, 1994, Journal of the National Cancer Institute, confirmed that silicone gel is carcinogenic in mice as well.

Supporting this experimental evidence, a 1989 FDA internal report stated: "A survey of the literature indicates numerous case reports of cancer" long after implantation and warned of the "possibility of worsened diagnosis" and prognosis when implanted women developed breast cancer. The report stressed that population studies claimed as proof of safety by industry and surgeons were too short-term and flawed to "negate the potential risk of cancer."

At known higher risk of breast cancer are 350,000 women with foam-wrapped implants. These consist of a silicone pouch wrapped in industrial polyurethane foam made from the carcinogenic synthetic petrochemical toluene diisocyanate (TDI). The foam is unstable in the body and breaks down into TDI and another carcinogen, TDA, which was removed from hair dyes in 1971 for that reason.

The foam-wrapped implants were developed to reduce scar-like hardening in some women following silicone implantation. However, their use beginning in the early 1980s ignored unequivocal evidence published two decades previously. Beginning in 1960, Wilhelm Hueper, the National Cancer Institute's leading carcinogenesis authority showed that foam degraded and induced malignant tumors in rats following injection and warned: "Since the polyurethane plastics have been used in cosmetic surgery . . . these observations are of practical importance . . . (and) should caution against indiscriminate use." He also noted that carcinogenic effects "might require an induction period of some 30 years or more," as with other carcinogens, notably asbestos. Hueper's finding have since been fully confirmed and extended by other independent studies.

Polyurethane-wrapped implants are thus carcinogen-impregnated sponges. These gradually disintegrate, releasing carcinogens to which the breast cells of premenopausal women are particularly sensitive.

Scientific publications apart, there is extensive documentation on industry's secret knowledge of cancer risks from implants, which were nevertheless aggressively marketed with assurances of safety. Dow Corning's carcinogenicity information on silicone implants is two decades old. Shortly after foam implants were first manufactured, the industry admitted that carcinogenicity data were "significant in those applications . . . for use inside the body." In 1985, Medical Engineering Corp., a Bristol-Myers Squibb subsidiary, admitted that "degradation products of polyurethane are toxic and in some cases carcinogenic. . . . Whether they are released in such low levels as to be no threat, only time will tell. . . . The breakdown products of the fuzzy implant material may well be carcinogenic. How would anyone defend himself in a malpractice suit if a patient developed a breast malignancy?" At industry-sponsored meetings in 1985, leading plastic surgeons cautioned that "foam could be a time bomb . . . (in view of its) carcinogenic potential. Surgeons should not go on implanting."

Without mentioning cancer risk, in April, 1992, the FDA banned all silicone implants except for controlled trials. This action was aggressively challenged by the American Society of Plastic and Reconstructive Surgery, the American College of Radiology and the American Medical Assn.

Responsibility for undisclosed cancer risks in 2 million implanted women, most seriously in the 350,000 with foam implants, is broadly shared among: the industry, for egregious conduct; plastic surgeons, for self-interested complicity; the FDA, for reckless unresponsiveness; the American Cancer Society, for silence, and the media, for minimal coverage of longstanding evidence. An immediate medical alert should be sent to all implanted women, with priority for those with foam implants. This should be followed by long-term surveillance with offers to remove the implants of any concerned women, at industry's but not taxpayers' expense. And all of this should be thoroughly apart from the inadequate $4.25-billion settlement.

October 26, 1997, *Chicago Tribune*

AWARENESS MONTH KEEPS WOMEN
PERILOUSLY UNAWARE

This October marks the 13th anniversary of the National Breast Cancer Awareness Month (NBCAM), with its flagship Oct. 17 National Mammography Day. Enthusiastically promoted by the "cancer establishment"—the American Cancer Society and the National Cancer Institute—the American College of Radiology and mainstream women's group, NBCAM is dedicated to reducing breast cancer mortality through early detection by mammography screening. With an estimated 180,000 new cases and 44,000 deaths in 1997—breast cancer is second only to lung cancer as the leading cause of cancer death in women—What could be a more worthy objective!

Unfortunately, the primary focus of NBCAM reveals profoundly misguided priorities and a disturbing lack of commitment to prevention. NBCAM is based on the insistence, exemplified by the American Cancer Society's statement in its "Cancer Facts and Figures—1997," that there are no "practical ways to prevent breast cancer. . . . Since women may not be able to alter their personal risk factors, the best opportunity for reducing mortality is through early detection" by mammography. Similarly, The National Cancer Institute's 1995 Special Presidential Commission on Breast Cancer maintained that breast cancer is "simply not a preventable disease," while requesting more funding for research on detection and treatment.

In fact the benefits of annual screening to women age 40 to 50, who are now being aggressively recruited, are at best controversial. In this age group, one in four cancers is missed at each mammography. Over a decade of premenopausal screening, as many as three in 10 women will be mistakenly diagnosed with breast cancer. Moreover, international studies have shown that routine premenopausal mammography is associated with increased breast cancer death rates at older ages. Factors involved include: the high sensitivity of the premenopausal breast to the cumulative carcinogenic effects of mammographic X-radiation; the still higher sensitivity to radiation of women who carry the A-T gene; and the danger that forceful and often painful compression of the breast during mammography may rupture small blood vessels and encourage distant spread of undetected cancers.

Apart from the dangers and questionable value of premenopausal screening is its apparently unrecognized and prohibitive cost of $2.5 billion annually—based on an average of $125 per mammogram for approximately 20 million US women age 40-50—which is more than the budgets of the National Cancer Institute and American Cancer Society combined.

While the benefits of postmenopausal screening are less controversial, there is little evidence that the usual US overkill of taking four or more mammograms per breast annually is any more effective than the more restrained European practice of a single view every two to three years. Furthermore, there is no evidence that screening at any age is more effective than monthly breast self-examination, especially by women trained in this procedure, combined with an annual clinical examination whose costs are minimal.

Underlying this indifference to prevention are interlocking conflicts of interest between the cancer establishment and the cancer drug industry, and between the American Cancer Society and American College of Radiology and the powerful mammography machine and film industries. More significantly, NBCAM was conceived and funded in 1984 by Imperial Chemical Industries, one of the world's largest petrochemical manufacturers, and its US subsidiary and spinoff Zeneca Pharmaceuticals.

Zeneca is the sole manufacturer of tamoxifen, the world's top-selling cancer drug, widely used for treating breast cancer and also for ill-advised trials to see whether it can prevent the disease in healthy women even though it is itself strongly carcinogenic. Of further concern, Zeneca has recently acquired 11 major cancer centers from Salick Health Care, posing disturbing and precedent-setting conflicts of interest between drug manufacture and prescription. Financial sponsorship by Zeneca gives it editorial control over every leaflet, poster, publication and commercial produced by NBCAM. As such, NBCAM is a masterful public relations coup for Zeneca.

With this background, it is hardly surprising that NBCAM fails to inform women how they can reduce their risks of breast cancer. In fact, we know a great deal about its avoidable causes, which include:

- Prolonged use of oral contraceptives and estrogen replacement therapy.
- High-fat animal and dairy product diets that are heavily contaminated with chlorinated pesticides that are estrogenic and carcinogenic to the breast, and meat contaminated with potent sex hormones following their use to fatten cattle in feed lots prior to slaughter.
- Exposure to petrochemical carcinogens in the workplace that put about 1 million US women at increased risk.
- Exposure to carcinogenic chemicals from hazardous waste sites and petrochemical plants that pollute soil, air and water.
- Exposure to indoor air pollutants, including, carcinogenic pesticides and solvents.
- Prolonged use of black and dark brown permanent or semi-permanent hair dyes.

- Heavy smoking and drinking commencing in adolescence,
- Inactivity and obesity.

Making women aware of these avoidable risks rather than fixating just on early detection should be the goal of a truly effective National Breast Cancer Awareness Month.

April 19, 1998, *Chicago Tribune*

FAILURE TO FULLY DOCUMENT RISKS OF OSTEOPOROSIS DRUG IS "RECKLESS"

Eli Lilly recently began running full-page color ads for Evista, a synthetic hormone with both estrogenic and antiestrogenic effects, in major national and regional newspaper's Tile ads claim that Evista offers "a new way to prevent osteoporosis," but at the same time admit that "its effect on fractures is not yet known." The ads also claim that women taking Evista had no increased *risks* of breast and uterine cancers, in contrast to conventional hormone replacement therapy, and that it reduces LDL or bad cholesterol blood levels. This should be welcome news to women worldwide particularly as osteoporosis has now reached epidemic proportions, affecting 15 million to 20 million American women each year; osteoporosis causes more than a million fractures, including 250.000 hip fractures, and kills some 50,000 elderly women, from complications as a result of their fractures.

While warning of some possible side effects, such as blood clots or hot flashes, Lilly fails to warn of the more serious risks of ovarian cancer. A company sponsored article in the Dec. 4, 1997 issue of The New England Journal of Medicine also ignores this risk. Lilly's pre-market clearance study, however, clearly shows that Evista induces ovarian cancer in both mice and rats. Furthermore, carcinogenic effects were noted at dosages well below the recommended therapeutic level. However, the study concluded: "The clinical relevance of these tumor findings is not known." Lilly reached this conclusion despite the strong scientific consensus that the induction of cancer in well designed tests in two rodent species creates the strong presumption of human risk. Nevertheless, Lilly fails to disclose this critical information in its ads and in its "warning" to patients.

Responding to such criticisms by one of us (Samuel Epstein) during a broadcast of the "Jim Lehrer Newshour" earlier this year [Jan. 12], a Lilly spokesman claimed that the carcinogenic effects of Evista in the ovaries of sexually mature rodents are irrelevant to such risks in postmenopausal women, as their ovaries are inactive, and, therefore, no warning is necessary, apart from the fact that the rodent studies were specifically designed to evaluate Evista's safety. Ovarian cancer is a scientifically documented complication of long term estrogen replacement therapy in post-menopausal women. Also disturbing is the claim that Evista poses no risks of breast and uterine cancers, based on clinical trials over only some 40 months, a period totally inadequate to possibly measure any such risks.

Ovarian cancer strikes about 24,000 women in the United States every year, accounting for 4 percent of all female cancers. About 15,000 women die annually from ovarian cancer, making it the most lethal of all female reproductive cancers. Lilly's suppression of its own evidence of ovarian cancer risks from Evista is reckless and threatening to women's health and life. Equally reckless is the Food and Drug Administration's December 1997 marketing clearance, especially in the absence of any requirement for warning. Such conduct clearly merits urgent congressional investigation, Evista should be withdrawn from the world market immediately. As importantly, a "cancer alert" should be sent to the more than 12,000 women who have participated in US and international clinical trials, in the absence of fully informed consent. The doctrine of informed consent is ethically and legally protective only when all facts relevant to benefits and risks are affirmatively disclosed. This is clearly not the case with women who have been involved in the Evista trials. These women should be offered semi-annual lifelong surveillance for the early detection of ovarian cancer at Eli Lilly's expense.

June 5, 1998, Chicago Tribune

NO SAFETY IN THESE IMPLANT NUMBERS

The *Tribune* editorial "seeking shelter from a legal storm" (May 22) on Dow Corning's decision to file for bankruptcy is misleading in the extreme.

The Tribune implies that women are lying about health problems they have suffered from silicone-gel breast implants and openly ignores efforts by Dow Corning to suppress its own evidence on the cancer risks of implants.

In a routine, August 1987 inspection, the Food and Drug Administration discovered the previously unreported results of a Dow Corning carcinogenicity test on the silicone gel used in its implants. Injection under the skin of rats induced a high incidence of malignant tumors. While Dow attempted to trivialize these findings by claiming that these cancers were non-specific "solid state tumors," this claim was dismissed by an FDA task force on grounds that these cancers were highly lethal, invaded distant organs and showed no variation in the incidence between male and female rates.

On the basis of these findings, a senior task-force scientist urged that a medical alert be issued to warn the public of the possibility of malignancy developing in humans following long-term implants or silicone breast prostheses. A July 1994 report by a National Cancer Institute investigator subsequently confirmed that silicone gel is also carcinogenic in mice.

At still higher risk of cancer are some 350,000 women with silicone implants wrapped in industrial-grade polyurethane foam. Evidence on the carcinogenicity of polyurethane was clearly demonstrated in the early 1960's. Subsequent studies showed that the foam breaks down in the breast to other carcinogens, toluene diisocyanate (TDI) and toluene diamine (TDA), which also induce breast cancer in rodents. (TDA was removed from hair dyes by the cosmetic industry in 1971 on the grounds of its carcinogenicity.)

Population studies, claimed as proof of safety by Dow and other implant manufacturers, are too short-term and otherwise flawed to negate the risk of cancer in some 2 million implanted women. Indeed, such studies would have exculpated asbestos in addition to most other recognized carcinogens, which have latencies extending over three decades. The study cited most often by industry as evidence of implants' safety was largely funded by plastic surgeons, who clearly have a vested interest in breast implants.

Rather than persisting in its egregious cover-up of the cancer risk of breast implants, apart from recent efforts to file for Chapter 11 to escape liability in breast-implant litigation, Dow Corning should immediately warn all implant women of their cancer risks, offer to remove their implants and develop long-term cancer surveillance at its own expense.

March 14, 2001, *Chicago Tribune*
MAMMOGRAPHY'S MIXED BLESSINGS

Mammography centers nationwide are scaling down or even closing because of inadequate Medicare payments and concerns about possible malpractice suits. While access to mammography is shrinking, the demand is increasing in the wake of aggressive promotion of premenopausal screening by the American Cancer Society.

Women now are waiting weeks or longer for appointments—potentially dangerous delays for those with lumps needing diagnostic mammography. With breast cancer on the increase—and now striking about 192,000 women and killing 41,000 annually—delayed detection promised by mammography surely poses a health care crisis. However, the crisis is more apparent than real, as screening is unreliable, dangerous—and inflationary.

- Mammography is not a technique for early diagnosis as breast cancer is rarely detectable until about eight years old.

- Evidence that screening allows early detection and treatment of breast cancer is tenuous based on analysis of two large trials, Danish researchers writing in the Lancet recently concluded: "There is no reliable evidence that screening decreases breast cancer mortality [and thus that] screening is unjustified."

- The Canadian National Breast Screening Study recently reported on a trial on some 39,000 postmenopausal women. Half of the women performed monthly breast self-examination, following instruction by trained nurses, had annual clinical breast examinations by trained nurses and also annual mammograms. The others practiced self-exams and had annual clinical exams but no mammograms. The authors of the study concluded that the mammographic detection of non-palpable cancers did not improve survival rates.

- False-negative mammograms are particularly common in premenopausal women because of their denser breast structure, and also in postmenopausal women on estrogen replacement therapy as some develop breast densities, making mammograms difficult to read.

- About one-third of all breast cancers and more still of the aggressive premenopausal cancers are discovered in the interval between successive annual mammograms. Premenopausal women particularly can thus be lulled into a false sense of security and fail to seek medical advice.

- False-positive mammograms, common in premenopausal and postmenopausal women on estrogen replacement therapy, result in needless anxiety, additional mammograms or unnecessary biopsies— even mastectomies. For some, the cumulative risk of false positives can reach as high as 100 percent over a decade of screening.

- Overdiagnosis is another risk. As screening becomes more common, pre-invasive breast ducts cancer, or ductal carcinoma-in-situ, is now diagnosed annually in some 40,000 women and often unnecessarily treated as invasive cancer by lumpectomy, plus radiation or even mastectomy. However, most of these pre-invasive cancers never become invasive, even if left untreated, and mortality is very low (1 percent)— the same for those diagnosed and treated early or late.

- Screening poses cumulative cancer risks. The routine of taking four films for each breast results in 1 rad (radiation absorbed dose) exposure, about 1,000 times more than a chest X-ray. The premenopausal breast is sensitive to radiation, each rad exposure increasing risk by 1 percent with a cumulative 10 percent increased risk over 10 years of screening; risks are greater for "baseline" screening at younger ages. Less well recognized dangers are posed by forceful breast compression during premenopausal mammography, which may rupture blood vessels in or around small undetected cancers and result in the spread of malignant cells.

- Finally, screening is inflationary; average Medicare and insurance costs are $70 and $125, respectively. If all 20 million premenopausal women had annual mammograms, minimum aggregate costs would be $2.5 billion; costs would reach $10 billion if the industry succeeds in replacing film machines, costing about $100,000, with digital machines, costing about $400,000, for which there is no evidence of improved effectiveness.

The combination of clinical exams and self-exams is effective, safe and low cost, unlike mammography. In 1985, ACS admitted: "At least 90 percent of the women who develop breast carcinoma discover the tumor themselves."

Nevertheless, the National Cancer Institute and the ACS, with ties to the American College of Radiology, and the mammography industry remain dismissive of breast examination as an alternative to mammography. National networks of clinical exam and self-exam clinics staffed by trained nurses should be established. These clinics would further empower women by providing scientific information on breast cancer prevention, of which women remain largely unaware.

ENDORSER:
Barbara Seaman
Co-Founder
National Women's Health Network
Washington, D.C.

February 25, 2002, *Los Angeles Times*
MAMMOGRAPHY DOESN'T COME WITHOUT RISK

The updated federal guidelines announced by Health and Human Services Secretary Tommy Thompson on Thursday strongly recommending annual screening mammography for women over the age of 40 are unlikely to resolve the current debate. The guidelines, surprisingly based on an unpublished analysis by an independent advisory board, ignore evidence on the risks of breast cancer from mammography.

Furthermore, they dismiss evidence on the effectiveness of monthly breast self-examination combined with annual clinical breast examination by trained health care professionals. None of these concerns are relevant to diagnostic mammography, the value of which is unchallenged.

Screening mammography poses significant and cumulative risks of radiation, particularly for premenopausal women. The routine practice of taking four films of each breast annually results in approximately 1 rad (radiation absorbed dose) exposure. This is about 1,000 times greater than exposure from a chest X-ray, which is broadly focused on the entire chest rather than narrowly on the breast. The premenopausal breast is highly sensitive to radiation, each 1 rad exposure increasing breast cancer risk by about 1%, with a cumulative 10% increased risk for each breast over a decade's screening.

Radiation risks are further increased fourfold for the 1% to 2% of women who are unknowing silent carriers of the A-T (ataxia-telangiectasia) gene. By some estimates, this accounts for up to 20% of all breast cancers diagnosed annually.

All these risks are greater for women in their 30s, who are being encouraged to undergo "baseline screening," for which there is no evidence of any future relevance.

Since 1928, physicians have been warned to handle cancerous breasts with care, for fear of accidentally disseminating cells and spreading the cancer. Mammography entails tight and often painful breast compression, particularly in premenopausal women. This may lead to the lethal spread of malignant cells by rupturing small blood vessels in or around small undetected breast cancers.

Another serious danger of mammography is the fact that mammography centers are being overbooked as a result of the aggressive promotion of premenopausal screening. Patients referred for diagnostic mammography because of suspicious clinical or other findings are now experiencing potentially life-threatening delays of up to several months before they can be examined.

The advisory panel's dismissal of self-examination and clinical examination is inconsistent with the results of a September 2000 publication by leading University of Toronto epidemiologists. Based on study of breast cancer mortality in 40,000 women, it was concluded that monthly self-examinations following brief training coupled with an annual examination by a trained health care professional is at least as effective as screening mammography in detecting small tumors.

National networks of clinics staffed by nurses trained in teaching monthly self-examination and conducting annual clinical examination should be established to replace mammography screening. Apart from their minimal costs, such clinics would empower women and free them from increasing dependence on industrialized medicine and complicit medical institutions.

It should be further pointed out that the new federal guidelines ignore the

. growing and inflationary costs of mammography. Screening all premenopausal women, 20 million annually, would cost about $2.5 billion. That is
equal to 14% of estimated Medicare spending on prescription drugs. These
costs would be increased fourfold if the highly profitable machine and film
industries succeed in replacing film machines, which cost about $100,000
each, with the latest high-tech digital machines, which cost about $400,000
each. The latter have been approved by the Food and Drug Administration
although there is no evidence of improved effectiveness.

CHAPTER 5

Press Releases & Huffington Post
Blog Posts, 1992–2011

February 4, 1992	The Push for Mammography May Be Off Target
March 2, 1993	The Cancer Establishment Ignores Avoidable Causes of Breast Cancer: Need for Initiatives by the New York City Commission on the Status of Women and by WEDO
February 22, 1994	Notice of Presentation: American Association for the Advancement of Science (AAAS), St. Francis Hilton, San Francisco
June 9, 1994	The Cancer Prevention Coalition Calls for the Replacement of the National Cancer Institute Director
October 18, 1994	National Mammoscam Day
May 11, 1995	Cancer Expert Calls Dow Breast Implant Ads Deceptive
October 18, 1995	National Mammography Day
November 8, 1995	New Study Warns Implants Pose Risk of Breast Cancer
February 2, 1998	New Challenges on the Safety of U.S. Meat: Oprah Right for Other Reasons
February 22, 1998	Major Cosmetic and Toiletry Ingredient Poses Avoidable Cancer Risks
March 30, 1998	Risk Factors: Hormonal Milk Poses Prostate Cancer and Other Cancer Risks
June 21, 1998	Monsanto's Hormonal Milk Poses Serious Risks of Breast Cancer, Besides Other Cancers
September 1, 1998	FDA Advisory Committee Urged to Reject Zeneca's Application of Tamoxifen for Preventing Breast Cancer in Healthy Women as the Drug is Ineffective and Dangerous
January 27, 1999	Misleading Claims by an Industry-Sponsored Study on the Safety of the Pill
March 7, 1999	Human Growth Hormone Anti-Aging Medication Poses Undisclosed Cancer Risks
May 3, 2001	The National Breast Cancer Coalition is Urged by Dr. Epstein to Consider Breast Examination as a Practical Alternative to Mammography
Febrary 6, 2002	Mammography is Dangerous Besides Ineffective
May 19, 2003	Genetically-Engineered Anti-Aging Medication, Monsanto Milk are Major, Unrecognized Risks of Breast Cancer
May 23, 2003	The American Cancer Society Misleads the Public
November 4, 2003	An Ounce of Prevention
October 28, 2005	The Look Good...Feel Better Program: But at What Risk?
June 27, 2006	Hormonal Milk Poses Greater Risks than Just Twinning
April 2, 2007	The United Nations Takes the Initiative in the War Against Cancer
May 16, 2007	Avoidable Causes of Breast Cancer
October 16, 2007	The Breast Cancer Awareness Mont Misleads Women
June 15, 2009	Medical Experts Prescribe Legislation to Help Prevent Cancer
October 8, 2009	Unrecognized Cancer and Hormonal Risks of Avon Products

November 17, 2009   UK Leads the Way in Banning Toxic Ingredients in
                    Cosmetics and Personal Care Products
November 24, 2009   Risks of Mammography: Hidden Role of the American
                    Cancer Society
December 16, 2009   HUFFINGTON POST: Reckless Indifference of the
                    American Cancer Society to Cancer Prevention
January 15, 2010   An FDA Ban on Genetically-Engineered Milk is Twenty
                    Years Overdue
February 25, 2010   HUFFINGTON POST: FDA Admits Medical Radiation
                    Risks, Ignores Mammography Dangers
March 29, 2010   Frank Conflicts of Interes in the National Cancer Institute
May 4, 2010   CPC Urged Support of the Safe Chemicals Act
May 7, 2010   Protect Children's Health from Toxic Bisphenol-A (BPA)
May 7, 2010   American Cancer Society Trivializes Cancer Risks: Blatant
                    Conflicts of Interest
June 16, 2010   Reckless Failure of the US Food and Drug Administration
                    to Protect Against Cancer from Toxics in Cosmetics and
                    GE Milk
October 15, 2010   HUFFINGTON POST: Breast Cancer *Unawareness* Month:
                    Rethinking Mammograms
January 10, 2011   Unrecognized Dangers of Formaldehyde
March 14, 2011   The American Cancer Society: "More Interested in
                    Accumulating Wealth than Saving Lives"
October 21, 2011   Corporate Sponsors Control Mammography Industry
October 28, 2011   National Mammography Day
December 9, 2011   Why We are Still Losing the Winnable War Against Cancer

February 4, 1992

THE PUSH FOR MAMMOGRAPHY MAY BE OFF TARGET

The Breast Cancer Coalition, a grass-roots group of women's consumer-health and provider organizations and the American Cancer Society, is holding hearings in Washington Wednesday to focus on the breast cancer epidemic now striking one in nine women.

Last year, the Coalition succeeded in increasing the National Cancer Institute's budget by $30 million for research into causes, screening and treatment of breast cancer. The Coalition is pressing for even more NCI funds, and it has been co-opted into supporting discredited policies of the lavishly funded cancer establishment.

The cancer establishment—NCI and American Cancer Society—concentrates on basic research, diagnosis and treatment. Cancer cause and prevention net only about 5% of the $1.8 billion annual NCI budget. The establishment is also closely interlocked with giant pharmaceutical firms whose cancer-drug sales net $1 billion annually.

Neither the establishment nor the coalition has recognized that the increase in breast cancer incidence, 57% since 1950, is similar to or less than the increases for other cancers: 44% for all cancer, 60% for male colon cancer, 100% for testis, prostate and kidney cancer, over 100%.

Also, unrecognized is mounting evidence relating cancer increased breast cancer to avoidable contamination of food, air and water and the workplace with industrial carcinogens and radiation.

The establishment, with Coalition support, is pushing for more mammography facilities. But the General Accounting Office reports, "there are more than enough machines to meet screening needs."

The establishment is also pushing for annual mammograms over age 40. There is general agreement that mammography improves cancer detection and survival in postmenopausal women, especially in modern facilities. But there is no evidence of benefit for younger women in whom screening, especially with X-ray exposures common on the '70's, caused more cancers than detected.

These concerns are emphasized by a recent Canadian study reporting 50% increased breast cancer mortality in women over 40 given annual mammograms vs. those given physical examinations only. Other studies have confirmed the dangers of routine mammograms in pre-menopausal women.

In spite of such evidence since the '60's, women have never been warned of mammography risks. The reasons may be explained by a confidential memo from an NCI physician in charge of large-scale NCI and ACS screening in 1973. These programs, he confided, "will gain [us] a great deal of favorable publicity –and will assist in obtaining more research funds."

The Breast Cancer Coalition needs to rethink its policies on mammograms. Screening young women should be abandoned. Obsolete high-dose equipment should be banned, as should untrained mammogram entrepreneurs. The role of past mammography in increasing cancer rates must be admitted and investigated. Women must be informed of their X-ray dosage from each screening and warned of the cancer risk.

Apart from physical examination, safe alternatives to mammography, particularly transillumination with infrared light scanning, should be developed and made available on a crash basis.

The cancer establishment insists that fatty diet itself is a major cause of breast cancer, although proof for this is minimal at best. There is, instead, growing evidence of the role of carcinogenic pesticides and other contaminants in fat, such as DDT and PCBs which accumulate in the breast and which mimic the hormonal effects of estrogens. A related risk if lifelong exposure to estrogenic contaminants in dietary fat from their unregulated use of growth-promoting cattle-feed additives.

Public health is too important to be left to self-interested establishment professional and politicized bureaucracies. But to be effective, grass-roots advocacy requires radical new thinking besides good intentions.

The Coalition should heed today's Washington Press conference, representing 60-plus prominent scientists who demand a total overhaul of federal cancer policies and who charge the cancer establishment with disinterest in cancer prevention and with misleading the nation into believing that we are "winning the war against cancer" while the facts show the contrary to be the case.

March 2, 1993

THE CANCER ESTABLISHMENT IGNORES AVOIDABLE CAUSES OF BREAST CANCER: NEED FOR INITIATIVES BY THE NEW YORK CITY COMMISSION ON THE STATUS OF WOMEN AND BY WEDO

Despite expenditures of over $1 billion on breast cancer over the last two decades, "we must conclude that there has been no progress in preventing the disease." The cancer establishment, the National Cancer Institute (NCI) and American Cancer Society (ACS), has long been, and still is, fixated on diagnosis and treatment and indifferent to or ignorant of cancer prevention. Establishment programs on breast cancer prevention reflect myopia and questionable science, as illustrated by their unsupported emphasis on high fat diet as the major cause. This is compounded by neglect of or unfamiliarity with longstanding evidence incriminating a wide range of environmental causes, particularly avoidable exposures to chemical and radioactive carcinogens (notably large scale emissions and discharges from civilian nuclear reactors) in air, water, food, and the workplace. Equally alarming is the cancer establishment's exploitation of women as scientific quinea pigs as evidenced by: their deliberate exposure of some 300,000 women without warning to high dose mammography in the 1970's; their failure to warn against breast cancer risks of the injectable contraceptive Depo-Provera; and by the grave risks of their ill-conceived breast cancer prevention trial with the carcinogenic drug tamoxifen.

CARCINOGENIC DIETARY CONTAMINANTS

None of the cancer establishment's heavily funded nutritional studies claiming associations between dietary fat and breast cancer (besides colon and other cancers) have investigated or even considered the role of carcinogenic dietary contaminants. Evidence for their role has accumulated over the last two decades and includes the following:

- Carcinogenic organocholrine pesticides, such as DDT, chlordane and dieldrin, which concentrate in animal fats, induce breast cancer in rodents. This creates the strong presumption for a causal role of such dietary contaminants in human breast cancer, particularly as the sites of cancer induced by carcinogens are generally similar in experimental animals and humans.
- Promotion by DDT of breast cancers induced in rodents by the potent carcinogen acetamidophenanthrene.
- DDT and PCBs concentrate in human breast cancer itself in contrast to adjacent non-cancerous tissue, and also in breasts with cancer in contrast to those with fibrocystic disease.
- Breast cancer mortality in premenopausal Israeli women declined by 30 percent following regulations in the mid 1970's reducing levels of DDT and other carcinogenic organochlorine pesticides in dietary fat, in spite of increasing fat consumption and decreasing birth rates.
- In view of the known carcinogenicity of exogenous estrogens, lifelong exposure to estrogenic contaminants in meat due to their unregulated use as growth-promoting feed additives, is clearly a risk factor for breast cancer. Warnings of such risks, including by Dr. Roy Hertz NCI's former leading expert in endocrinology, have gone unheeded.
- Exogenous estrogens synergize the carcinogenic effects of irradiation, and also of polynuclear hydrocarbon carcinogens in the rodent breast.

It may be further noted that the cancer establishment remained silent while the Bush Administration revoked the 1958 Delaney law banning the deliberate contamination of processed foods with carcinogenic pesticides.

MAMMOGRAPHY

While there is general consensus that mammography improves early cancer detection and survival in post menopausal women, no such benefits have been demonstrated for younger women. Additionally, there is clear evidence that the breast, particularly in pre-menopausal women, is highly sensitive to the carcinogenic effects of radiation. Although this was well known since the late 1960's, the NCI and ACS embarked on a large scale Breast Cancer Detection Demonstration Program using high radiation exposures which, as admitted by a senior NCI epidemiologist then involved in the program, were likely to cause more breast cancers than could be detected. These concerns persist today, even with lower level radiation exposure. This is evidenced by several studies which show excess breast cancer mortality in pre-menopausal women receiving repeated mammograms. Available scientific information justifies the following recommendations:

- Pressures for expansion of the mammography industry should be strongly resisted, especially in view of the conclusion that "there are more than enough machines to meet the screening needs of American women."
- Mammography should be restricted to post-menopausal women.
- Mammography should be conducted only in major medical centeres with licensed technicians using dedicated equipment calibrated at regular intervals.
- Women should be provided with information on actual, not just estimated, radiation doses at each mammography.
- The use of mammography should be phased out. Crash programs should be developed to develop and make available safe and similarly effective screening procedures, particularly transillumination with infrared light scanning.

It should further be stressed that the carcinogenic effects of "low dose" radiation are disproportionately greater than those from a single cumulative equivalent large dose exposure, and also that a significant proportion of the general population have high genetic sensitivity to radiation-induced breast cancer.

DEPO-PROVERA

Depo-Provera (DP) is a synthetic progesterone given by injection for long term contraception. Its use was approved by the Bush administration's Food and Drug Administration (FDA) in June 1992 in spite of unequivocal evidence of its carcinogenicity. DP induces breast cancer in mice and dogs. This evidence has been confirmed by recent international epidemiological studies demonstration high risks of breast cancer, particularly when DP's use is started before the age of 20 and continued for over two years. Other complications, include osteoporosis, depression, loss of libido, and substantial weight gain. Incredibly, the NCI and ACS have remained silent while this new major breast cancer risk has been introduced in the US.

Based on experience abroad, there seems little doubt that this dangerous contraceptive will be selectively offered to low income ethnic minority groups, just those women with the least power and most easily coerced.

THE TAMOXIFEN TRIAL

In spring 1992, the NCI embarked on a large scale breast cancer trial recruiting thousands of healthy women at increased risk of breast cancer, including those with close relatives with the disease and also anyone over 60. Half these women are being treated with tamoxifen, a drug closely related to DES, while the rest receive a placebo. NCI claims that tamoxifen can reduce breast cancer by 30%, while also reducing heart attacks and preventing osteoporosis.

Not only is there no scientific basis for the alleged benefits of tamoxifen, but there is also substantial evidence of its grave risks of liver ad uterus cancer, besides a wide range of other toxic effects. Any oncologist or institute participating in these trials is at serious risk of future malpractice and punitive claims.

THE ROLE OF NEW YORK CITY COMMISSION AND WEDO

It is recommended that the Commission and WEDO set up a series of task forces to investigate the following: the failure of the cancer establishment to undertake programs on breast cancer prevention; their failure to warn of avoidable causes of breast cancer; their failure to support available non-hazardous alternatives to mammography; their silence on the carcinogenic hazards of Depo-Provera; and, the scientific and ethical travesty of their tamoxifen trial.

It is further recommended that the Commission and WEDO widely disseminate information relating escalating breast cancer rates to the overall current cancer epidemic now striking one in three and killing one in four. The involvement of activist women's groups should be extended to even broader concerns on cancer prevention in general.

It is finally recommended, that the Commission and WEDO join with the Cancer Prevention Coalition in appropriate and aggressive action to reform the policies and priorities of the NCI and ACS.

February 22, 1994
NOTICE OF PRESENTATION: AMERICAN ASSOCIATION FOR THE ADVANCEMENT OF SCIENCE (AAAS), ST. FRANCIS HILTON, SAN FRANCISCO

- Dr. Samuel S. Epstein condemns the cancer establishment—NCI and ACS—for overwhelming neglect of breast cancer prevention.
- Mounting evidence links women's breast cancer epidemic to avoidable carcinogenic exposures in food, the workplace & environment.
- Not only does the American Cancer Society (ACS) neglect prevention, it recklessly promotes premenopausal mammography, despite its ineffectiveness and excess risk of breast cancer deaths.
- While failing to pursue prevention, the cancer establishment has embarked on Orwellian experiments exposing healthy women to the carcinogenic drug, tamoxifen, which is very likely to cause, rather than prevent, more cancer.
- A new breast cancer risk is women's exposure to the milk from rBGH-

treated cows, which contains sustained, elevated levels of IGF-1, a potent growth factor.

Dr. Samuel S. Epstein, the chairman of the Cancer Prevention Coalition, condemns the cancer establishment for its overwhelming neglect of cancer prevention, especially the prevention of women's breast cancer.

Risks that could be avoided are being ignored by the cancer establishment—the National Cancer Institute (NCI) and the American Cancer Society (ACS)—despite their expenditures of more than $1 billion dollars on breast cancer research.

Accumulating evidence links the growing epidemic of women's breast cancer to exposure to avoidable carcinogens in the diet, the workplace and the general environment.

Such avoidable risks include carcinogenic and estrogenic food contaminants, particularly pesticides, some of which induce breast cancer in experimental animals; exposures to known mammary carcinogens in the workplace; and radiation, particularly pre-menopausal mammography.

Dr. Epstein stated, "Instead of promoting prevention, the American Cancer Society is recklessly promoting premenopausal mammography, despite its ineffectiveness and its excess risk of breast cancer deaths."

Dr. Epstein added, "While failing to pursue cancer prevention, the cancer establishment has embarked on Orwellian chemoprevention experiments exposing healthy women to the highly carcinogenic tamoxifen, manufactured by Zeneca Pharmaceuticals. Such treatment is likely to cause more uterine and other cancers, rather than prevent breast cancer. An even more bizarre attempt at breast cancer prevention is the administration of hormonal cocktails designed to block 'incessant ovulation' in healthy young women."

Continued Dr. Epstein, "All women from conception to death will now be exposed to an additional breast cancer risk, the milk from cows treated with recombinant bovine growth hormone (rBGH). Milk from cows injected with this Monsanto drug contains sustained, elevated levels of IGF-1, a potent growth factor which is a potential causes of breast cancer."

Dr. Epstein concluded, "It's time for radical reforms in the leadership and priorities of both the National Cancer Institute and the American Cancer Society, in view of their longstanding, overwhelming neglect of cancer prevention by reducing avoidable exposures to industrial and other carcinogens in air, water, food, and the workplace."

June 9, 1994
THE CANCER PREVENTION COALITION CALLS FOR THE REPLACEMENT OF THE NATIONAL CANCER INSTITUTE DIRECTOR

In a letter sent today to President Clinton, the Cancer Prevention Coalition (CPC), a nation-wide coalition of cancer prevention experts, and citizen activists, calls for the immediate replacement of Dr. Samuel Broder, director of the National Cancer Institute (NCI).

According to Dr. Samuel Epstein, Chairman of CPC, "Dr. Broder has recently attempted to distance himself from serious scientific fraud, involving NCI breast cancer treatment trials, coordinated by University of Pittsburgh's Dr. Fisher. However, clear evidence of this fraud, involving taxpayers' dollars, was well known some three years ago to Dr. Broder who failed to take any corrective action, let alone inform cancer patients. Furthermore, NCI has embarked on a breast cancer 'prevention' trial on healthy women treated with tamoxifen, also coordinated by Dr. Fisher. NCI's prevention claims are scientifically questionable if not reckless, and the patient consent forms misleadingly trivialize serious toxic effects of the drug, including aggressive uterine and liver cancers."

Additionally, the CPC directors charge NCI "with having misled the public and Congress into believing that we are winning the war against cancer. In fact, we are losing this war. Cancer rates are escalating to epidemic proportions, now striking more than one in three and killing more than one in four. Also, our ability to treat and cure most cancers has not improved for decades. Moreover, the inflationary costs of cancer are a major factor in the current health care crisis. Meanwhile, NCI is indifferent if not hostile to cancer prevention."

The letter to the President details the following charges:

- NCI allocates less than 2.5% of its $2 billion annual budget to research on avoidable exposures to environmental and occupational carcinogens.

- NCI has been silent with regard to the contamination of hot dogs with the highly potent carcinogen dimethylnitrosamine, although this has been known since the early 1970's. A recent study links frequent hot dog consumption with childhood leukemia and brain cancer.
- The Institute has failed to warn some fifty million women who use permanent hair dyes of the risks of lymphomas and other cancers.

The Coalition concluded, "Dr. Broder's replacement by a qualified scientist with balanced interest in prevention, treatment and basic research is clearly overdue. But this is not enough. Radical reforms are needed to redirect NCI policies and priorities, with greater emphasis on cancer prevention by research informational and interventional programs."

October 18, 1994

NATIONAL MAMMOSCAM DAY

Commenting on tomorrow's National Mammography Day, Dr. Samuel Epstein, Chairman of the Cancer Prevention Coalition (CPC), charged that "this is a recklessly misleading and self-interested promotional event, more aptly named NATIONAL MAMMOSCAM DAY."

National Mammography Day, October 19, is the flagship of October's National Breast Cancer Awareness Month (NBCAM). NBCAM was conceived and funded in 1984 by Imperial Chemical Industries (ICI) and its US subsidiary and spinoff Zeneca Pharmaceuticals. NBCAM is a multi-million-dollar deal with the cancer establishment, the National Cancer Institute (NCI) and American Cancer Society (ACS) and its multiple corporate sponsors, and the American College of Radiology.

ICI is one of the largest manufacturers of petrochemical and organochlorines, and Zeneca is the sole manufacturer of tamoxifen, the world's top selling cancer drug widely used for breast cancer. Zeneca/ICI's financial sponsorship gives them control over every leaflet, poster, publication, and commercial produced by NBCAM.

ICI supports the NBCAM blame-the-victim theory of cancer causation, which attributes escalating rates of breast (and other) cancers to heredity and faulty lifestyle. This theory diverts attention away from avoidable exposures to carcinogenic industrial contaminants of air, water, food, consumer products, and the workplace—the same products which ICI has manufactured for decades. Ignoring prevention of breast cancer, NBCAM promotes "early" detection by mammography.

There are a wide range of serious problems with mammography, particularly with premenopausal women:

- There is no evidence of the effectiveness or benefit of mammography in pre-menopausal women.

- By the time breast cancers can be detected by mammography, they are up to 8 years old. By then, some will have spread to local lymph nodes or to distant organs, especially in younger women.

- Missed cancers (false negatives) are commonplace among younger women, as their dense breast tissues limit penetration by x-rays.

- About 1 in every 4 "tumors" identified by mammography in premenopausal women turns out not to be cancer following biopsy (false positive). Apart from needless anxiety, repeated surgery can result in scarring, and delayed identification of early cancer that may subsequently develop.

- Regular mammography of younger women increases their cancer risks, particularly for women already at risk for familial reasons. Analysis of controlled trials over the last decade, has shown consistent increases in breast cancer mortality within a few years of commencing screening. This confirms evidence on the high sensitivity of the pre-menopausal breast, and on cumulative carcinogenic effects of radiation.

- Pre-menopausal women carrying the A-T gene, about 1.5 percent of women, are more radiation sensitive and at higher cancer risk from mammography. It has been estimated that up to 10,000 breast cancer cases each year are due to mammography of A-T carriers.

- Radiation, particularly from repeated pre-menopausal mammography, is likely to interact additively or synergistically with other avoidable causes of breast cancer, particularly estrogens (natural; medical; contaminants of meat from cattle feed additives; and estrogenic pesticides).

- Forceful compression of the breast during mammography, particularly in younger women, may cause the spread of small undetected cancers.

Pressured by this evidence on the ineffectiveness and risks of pre-menopausal mammography, NCI recently withdrew recommendations for such screening. This evidence is still ignored by NBCAM, supported by radiologists and giant mammography machine and film corporations, which has specifically targeted pre-menopausal women with high-pressured advertisements.

CPC urges the immediate phase-out of pre-menopausal mammography. Post-menopausal mammography should be restricted to major centers and exposure reduced to a minimum. Women should be provided with actual close measurements, rather than estimates. NCI and ACS should develop large-scale use of safe screening alternatives, including imaging techniques, and blood or urine tumor markers or immunologic tests.

Dr. Epstein urges that a medical alert should be sent to women subjected to the Breast Cancer Detection Demonstration Project high dose radiation experiments commencing in 1972. These experiments were conducted in spite of explicit prior warnings by a National Academy of Sciences committee, and also by former senior NCI staffer, and noted epidemiologist, Dr. John Bailar. He cautioned, "Such radiation in pre-menopausal women would be likely to cause more breast cancers than could be detected." Dr. Bailar now concludes, "This experiment could well account for an "immediate investigation of the cancer establishment's reckless conduct by the President's Committee on Human Radiation Experiments."

ENDORSER:
Dr. John Bailar
Professor of Epidemiology and Biostatistics
McGill University
Montreal, Quebec, Canada

May 11, 1995
CANCER EXPERT CALLS DOW BREAST IMPLANT ADS DECEPTIVE

Dr. Samuel Epstein, Professor of Environmental and Occupational Medicine at the University of Illinois (at Chicago) School of Public Health and internationally recognized authority on cancer prevention, will present evidence, including an unpublished Dow study, on the cancer risks of silicone breast implants at the May 13 Silicone Device Conference.

"Recent Dow Corning advertisements on the safety of breast implants are deceptive in the extreme and are highly unethical," commented Dr. Epstein.

Dr. Epstein will offer a detailed critique of the Dow ads, in addition to a wide range of other evidence on the cancer risks of breast implants, at the conference to be held at 9:00 a.m. at the Washington Renaissance Hotel, 999 9th St. N.W. Washington, DC. He will charge the implant industry and government with a cover-up of these risks to some two million women. Highlights will include:

Unpublished Dow Corning studies discovered in a 1987 FDA inspection showed that silicone gel injection induced highly malignant tumors in rats. FDA scientists concluded in a confidential memorandum that: "While there is no direct proof that silicone causes cancer in humans, there is considerable evidence that it can do so." Accordingly, it was recommended that "a medical alert be issued to warn the public of the possibility of malignancy following long term implant(ation)."

A 1994 report in the Journal of the National Cancer Institute confirmed the carcinogenicity of silicone gel in experiments with mice.

A 1989 confidential FDA report admitted "numerous case reports of (breast) cancer" long after implantation. The report concluded that population studies, claimed as proof of safety by industry and plastic surgeons, are too short term and flawed to "negate the potential risk of cancer." The report also warned of the "possibility of worsened diagnosis" and prognosis when implanted women developed breast cancer. These conclusions were fully confirmed in a 1993 congressionally-mandated report by the National Cancer Institute (NCI).

Large scale use of foam-wrapped implants ignored evidence published in the early 1960's by NCI's leading authority on carcinogenesis, the late Dr. Wilhelm Hueper. Hueper's studies showed that foam gradually degrades and induces malignant tumors in rats. He warned: "Since the polyurethane plastics have been used in cosmetic surgery . . . these observations are of practical importance . . . (and) should caution against (their) indiscriminate use."

Over 350,000 women with silicone implants wrapped in industrial polyurethane foam to reduce scarring are at higher risk of cancer. Polyurethane foam is manufactured from the carcinogenic toluene diisocyanate (TDI) which breaks down into another carcinogen, TDA. It should be further noted that TDA was removed from hair dyes by the cosmetic industry in 1971 following discovery of its carcinogenicity.

In 1985, a Bristol-Myers subsidiary admitted that: "Degradation products of polyurethane are toxic and in some cases carcinogenic . . . The breakdown products of the fuzzy implant material may well be carcinogenic. How would anyone defend himself in a malpractice suit of a patient developed a breast malignancy."

At a 1985 industry-sponsored conference, a leading plastic surgeon cautioned that "foam could be a time bomb . . . (in view of its) carcinogenic potential. Surgeons should not go on implanting." Following identification of TDA in foam, a Bristol-Myers employee warned ". . . there is pretty solid evidence that (it) is a carcinogen. The question is does PU foam . . . release TDA in the human breast to an extent that causes an unacceptable risk of cancer."

Dr. Epstein will urge that the FDA issue a medical alert to all implanted women, with priority for those with foam implants. He also will urge that these women should be offered a program of comprehensive medical surveillance and be given the option of having their implants removed, both at industry's expense. "Dow Corning and other implant makers should be responsible for all costs," Dr. Epstein said.

ENDORSER:
Jill Stone
Founder
Triad Silicone Network

October 18, 1995
NATIONAL MAMMOGRAPHY DAY

Commenting on tomorrow's National Mammography Day, Dr. Samuel Epstein, Chairman of the Cancer Prevention Coalition (CPC), charged that "this is a recklessly misleading and self-interested promotional event, more aptly named NATIONAL MAMMOSCAM DAY."

National Mammography Day, October 19, is the flagship of October's National Breast Cancer Awareness Month (NBCAM). NBCAM was conceived and funded in 1984 by Imperial Chemical Industries (ICI) and its US subsidiary and spinoff Zeneca Pharmaceuticals. NBCAM is a multi-million-dollar deal with the cancer establishment, the National Cancer Institute (NCI) and American Cancer Society (ACS) and its multiple corporate sponsors, and the American College of Radiology.

ICI is one of the largest manufacturers of petrochemical and organochlorines, and Zeneca is the sole manufacturer of tamoxifen, the world's top selling cancer drug widely used for breast cancer. Zeneca/ICI's financial sponsorship gives them control over every leaflet, poster, publication, and commercial produced by NBCAM.

ICI supports the NBCAM blame-the-victim theory of cancer causation, which attributes escalating rates of breast (and other) cancers to heredity and faulty lifestyle. This theory diverts attention away from avoidable exposures to carcinogenic industrial contaminants of air, water, food, consumer products, and the workplace—the same products which ICI has manufactured for decades. Ignoring prevention of breast cancer, NBCAM promotes "early" detection by mammography.

There are a wide range of serious problems with mammography, particularly with premenopausal women:

- There is no evidence of the effectiveness or benefit of mammography in pre-menopausal women.
- By the time breast cancers can be detected by mammography, they are up to 8 years old. By then, some will have spread to local lymph nodes or to distant organs, especially in younger women.
- Missed cancers (false negatives) are commonplace among younger women, as their dense breast tissues limit penetration by x-rays.
- About 1 in every 4 "tumors" identified by mammography in premenopausal women turns out not to be cancer following biopsy (false positive). Apart from needless anxiety, repeated surgery can result in scarring, and delayed identification of early cancer that may subsequently develop.
- Regular mammography of younger women increases their cancer risks, particularly for women already at risk for familial reasons. Analysis of

controlled trials over the last decade, has shown consistent increases in breast cancer mortality within a few years of commencing screening. This confirms evidence on the high sensitivity of the pre-menopausal breast, and on cumulative carcinogenic effects of radiation.

- Pre-menopausal women carrying the A-T gene, about 1.5 percent of women, are more radiation sensitive and at higher cancer risk from mammography. It has been estimated that up to 10,000 breast cancer cases each year are due to mammography of A-T carriers.

- Radiation, particularly from repeated pre-menopausal mammography, is likely to interact additively or synergistically with other avoidable causes of breast cancer, particularly estrogens (natural; medical; contaminants of meat from cattle feed additives; and estrogenic pesticides).

- Forceful compression of the breast during mammography, particularly in younger women, may cause the spread of small undetected cancers.

Pressured by this evidence on the ineffectiveness and risks of pre-menopausal mammography, NCI recently withdrew recommendations for such screening. This evidence is still ignored by NBCAM, supported by radiologists and giant mammography machine and film corporations, which has specifically targeted pre-menopausal women with high-pressured advertisements.

CPC urges the immediate phase-out of pre-menopausal mammography. Post-menopausal mammography should be restricted to major centers and exposure reduced to a minimum. Women should be provided with actual close measurements, rather than estimates. NCI and ACS should develop large-scale use of safe screening alternatives, including imaging techniques, and blood or urine tumor markers or immunologic tests.

Dr. Epstein urges that a medical alert should be sent to women subjected to the Breast Cancer Detection Demonstration Project high dose radiation experiments commencing in 1972. These experiments were conducted in spite of explicit prior warnings by a National Academy of Sciences committee. Finally, Dr. Epstein calls for an "immediate investigation of the cancer establishment's reckless conduct by the President's Committee on Human Radiation Experiments."

November 8, 1995

NEW STUDY WARNS IMPLANTS POSE RISK OF BREAST CANCER

In the first comprehensive review of the scientific literature, internationally-recognized cancer expert Samuel Epstein MD, concludes that implants pose significant risks of breast cancer. The study will appear in the November issue of the peer-reviewed International Journal of Occupational Medicine and Toxicology.

The review presents a detailed analysis of the scientific literature, and confidential industry and government documents on the carcinogenicity of silicone and polyurethane breast implants.

"Risks of breast cancer have been ignored in the current controversy over implants" stated Dr. Epstein, Chair of the Cancer Prevention Coalition and pathology expert at the School of Public Health, University of Illinois-Chicago. "Evidence on the carcinogenicity of implants, particularly polyurethane, is strong. Recent epidemiological studies claimed as proof of safety are grossly flawed. Such studies would have even given a clean bill of health to asbestos."

Dr. Epstein continued, "Both industry and the Food and Drug Administration (FDA) have suppressed evidence on the cancer risk of silicone breast implants. FDA has still failed to act on the recommendation by their leading scientists to send Medical Alerts to women with silicone implants warning them of their cancer risks."

Based on his report, Dr. Epstein renews the call for a medical alert. He also urges the development of a long term surveillance program, at industry's expense, with priority for women with polyurethane implants.

February 2, 1998

NEW CHALLENGES ON THE SAFETY OF US MEAT: OPRAH RIGHT FOR OTHER REASONS

The World Trade Organization (WTO) ruled in favor of the 1989 European ban on the use of sex hormones for growth promotion of cattle in feedlots prior to slaughter. While subject to further assessment before it can be made permanent, this ruling is a major victory for European consumers. It is also a major defeat for the United States and Canada which challenged the European ban claiming that it was "protectionist," costing over $100 million a year in lost exports, and that it reflected "consumerism versus science." The WTO ruling also raises serious concerns on the safety of US meat, recently questioned on different grounds by Oprah Winfrey, based on the following considerations:

- Confidential industry reports to the FDA, obtained under the Freedom of Information Act, reveal high residues of natural and synthetic sex hormones in meat products even under ideal test conditions. This is contrary to repeated and explicit assurances by the FDA and USDA.

- Following legal implantation in the ear of steers of Synovex-S, a combination of estradiol and progesterone, estradiol levels in meat products ranged up to 20-fold in excess of the normal. Based on conservative estimates, the amount of estradiol in two hamburgers eaten by an 8-year-old boy could increase his hormone levels by 10%.

- Much higher hormone residues are found in meat products following illegal implantation in cattle muscle which is commonplace in US feedlots. The WTO ruled that such abuse alone would justify the European ban.

- Contrary to repeated and explicit assurances by the FDA and USDA, none of the approximately 130 million US livestock slaughtered annually are tested for residues of cancer-causing and gene-damaging estradiol or any related sex hormones. This misrepresentation has been confirmed by European Commission inspectors, in a November 1997 survey of US control programs, who reported that there was no monitoring for residues of sex hormones nor for illegal animal drugs, including antibiotics, and that US residue monitoring was totally inadequate to meet European standards.

- Repeated assurances on the safety of hormonal meat by two World Health Organization bodies, the Food and Agriculture Organization and the Codex Alimentarius Commission (FAO/CODEX), reflect minimal expertise in public health, high representation of senior FDA and USDA officials and industry consultants, reliance on unpublished industry and outdated scientific information, and conflicts of interest.

Paradoxically, the same Codex Commission which approved hormonal meat, explicitly warned over a decade ago that baby meat foods "shall be free from residues of hormones."

- The endocrine-disruptive effects of estrogenic pesticides and other industrial food contaminants, known as xenoestrogens, are now under intensive investigation by US regulatory and health agencies. But contamination of meat with residues of the thousands-fold more potent estradiol remains ignored.

- Lifelong exposure to high residues of natural and synthetic sex hormones in meat products poses serious risks of breast and other reproductive cancers, whose incidence in the US has sharply escalated since 1950—55% for breast cancer, 120% for testicular cancer, and 230% for prostate cancer. Those residues have also been incriminated in increasing trends of precocious sexual development.

Commenting on these facts, Samuel S. Epstein, M.D., Professor of Environmental Medicine at the University of Illinois Chicago, School of Public Health, stated: "The European ban on hormonal meat should serve as a long- overdue wake-up call for US consumers to demand an immediate ban on hormone use or, minimally, the explicit labeling of hormonal meat products. It should also lead to a congressional investigation of the FDA and USDA for gross regulatory abdication besides suppression of information vital to consumer health. The dangers of US hormonal meat can no longer be ignored."

February 22, 1998

MAJOR COSMETIC AND TOILETRY INGREDIENT POSES AVOIDABLE CANCER RISKS

As reported on CBS Morning News today, the National Toxicology Program (NTP) recently found that repeated skin application to mouse skin of diethanolamine (DEA), or its fatty acid derivative cocamide-DEA, induced liver and kidney cancer. Besides this "clear evidence of carcinogenicity," NTP also emphasized that DEA is readily absorbed through the skin and accumulates in organs, such as the brain, where it induces chronic toxic effects.

High concentrations of DEA-based detergents are commonly used in a wide range of cosmetics and toiletries, including shampoos, hair dyes and conditioners, lotions, creams and bubble baths, besides liquid dishwashing and laundry soaps. Lifelong use of these products thus clearly poses major avoidable cancer risks to the great majority of US consumers, particularly infants and young children.

Further increasing these cancer risks is longstanding evidence that DEA readily interacts with nitrite preservatives or contaminants in cosmetics or toiletries to form nitrosodiethanolamine (NDELA), another carcinogen as well recognized by Federal agencies and institutions and the World Health Organization, which, like DEA, is also rapidly absorbed through the skin. In 1979, FDA warned that over 40% of all cosmetic products were contaminated with NDELA and called for industry "to take immediate action to eliminate this carcinogen from cosmetic products." In two 1991 surveys, 27 out of 29 products were found to be contaminated with high concentrations of this carcinogen, results which were subsequently confirmed by the FDA. Based on this information, the European Union and European industry have both taken strong action to reduce or eliminate DEA and NDELA from cosmetics and toiletries. In sharp contrast, the FDA has taken no such action, nor has it responded to a 1996 petition from the Cancer Prevention Coalition to phase out the use of DEA or to label DEA-containing products with an explicit cancer warning. The mainstream US industry has been similarly unresponsive, even to the extent of ignoring an explicit warning by the Cosmetics, Toiletries and Fragrance Association to discontinue uses of DEA. Such reckless intransigence is in strong contrast to the responsiveness of the growing safe cosmetic industry.

Tom Mower, former CEO of Neways Inc., a major distributor of carcinogen-free cosmetics, emphasized: "I see no reason at all to use DEA, as there are safe and cost-effective alternatives which we have been using in a wide range of our cosmetics and toiletries for the last decade."

Faced with escalating cancer rates, now striking more than one in three Americans, FDA should take immediate action to prevent further exposure to the avoidable carcinogens DEA and NDELA in cosmetics, toiletries and liquid soaps. Safe and effective alternatives to DEA are readily available.

March 30, 1998

RISK FACTORS: HORMONAL MILK POSES RISKS OF PROSTATE AND OTHER CANCERS

As reported in a January 23, 1998 article in Science, men with high blood levels of the naturally occurring hormone insulin-like growth factor (IGF-1) are over four times more likely to develop [advanced] prostate cancer than are men with lower levels. The report emphasized that high IGF-1 blood levels are the strongest known risk factor for prostate cancer, only exceeding that of a family history, and that reducing IGF-1 levels is likely to prevent this cancer. It was further noted that IGF-1 markedly stimulates the division and proliferation of normal and cancerous prostate cells and that it blocks the programmed self-destruction of cancer cells thus enhancing the growth and invasiveness of latent prostate cancer. These findings are highly relevant to any efforts to prevent prostate cancer, whose rates have escalated by 180 percent since 1950, which is now the most common cancer in non-smoking men with an estimated 185,000 new cases and 39,000 deaths in 1998.

While warning that increasing IGF-1 blood levels by treating the elderly with growth hormone (GH) to slow aging may increase risks of prostate cancer, the 1998 report appears unaware of the fact that the entire US population is now exposed to high levels of IGF-1 in dairy products. In February 1995, the Food and Drug Administration approved the sale of unlabeled milk from cows injected with Monsanto's genetically engineered bovine growth hormone, rBGH, to increase milk production. As detailed in a January 1996 report in the International Journal of Health Services, rBGH milk differs from natural milk chemically, nutritionally, pharmacologically and immunologically, besides being contaminated with pus and antibiotics resulting from mastitis induced by the biotech hormone. Most critically, rBGH milk is supercharged with high levels of abnormally potent IGF-1, up to 10 times more potent. IGF-1 resists pasteurization and digestion by stomach enzymes and is well absorbed across the intestinal wall. Still unpublished Monsanto tests, disclosed by FDA in summary form in 1990, showed that statistically significant growth stimulating effects were induced in organs of adult rats by feeding IGF-1 levels and to increase risks of developing prostate cancer and promoting its invasiveness. Apart from prostate cancer, multiple lines of evidence have also incriminated the role of IGF-1 as risk factors for breast, colon, and childhood cancers.

Faced with escalating rates of prostate and other avoidable cancers, FDA should withdraw its approval of rBGH milk, whose sale benefits only Monsanto while posing major public health risks form the entire US population. Failing early FDA action, consumers should demand explicit labeling and only buy rBGH-free milk.

June 21, 1998

MONSANTO'S HORMONAL MILK POSES SERIOUS RISKS OF BREAST BESIDES OTHER CANCERS

As reported in a May 9 article in The Lancet, women with a relatively small increase in blood levels of the naturally occurring growth hormone Insulin-like Growth Factor I (IGF-1) are up to seven times more likely to develop premenopausal breast cancer than women with lower levels. Based on those results, the report concluded that the risks of elevated IGF-1 blood levels are among the leading known risk factors for breast cancer, and are exceeded only by a strong family history or unusual mammographic abnormalities. Apart from breast cancer, an accompanying editorial warned that elevated IGF-1 levels are also associated with greater than any known risk factors for other major cancers, particularly colon and prostate.

This latest evidence is not unexpected. Higher rates of breast, besides colon, cancer have been reported in patients with gigantism (acromegaly) who have high IGF-1 blood levels. Other studies have also shown that administration of IGF-1 to elderly female primates causes marked breast enlargement and proliferation of breast tissue, that IGF-1 is a potent stimulator of human breast cells in tissue culture, that it blocks the programmed self-destruction of breast cancer cells, and enhances their growth and invasiveness.

These various reports, however, appear surprisingly unaware of the fact that the entire US population is now exposed to high levels of IGF-1 in dairy products. In February 1995, the Food and Drug Administration approved the sale of unlabelled milk from cows injected with Monsanto's genetically engineered bovine growth hormone, rBGH, to increase milk production. As detailed in a January 1996 report in the prestigious *International Journal of Health Services*, rBGH milk differs from natural milk chemically, nutritionally, pharmacologically and immunologically, besides being contaminated with pus and antibiotics resulting from mastitis induced by the biotech hormone. More critically, rBGH milk is supercharged with high levels of abnormally potent IGF-1, up 10 times the levels in natural milk and over 10 times more potent. IGF-1 resists pasteurization, digestion by stomach enzymes, and is well absorbed across the intestinal wall. Still unpublished 1987 Monsanto tests, disclosed by FDA in summary form in 1990, revealed that statistically significant growth stimulating effects were induced in organs of adult rats by feeding IGF-1 at low dose levels for only two weeks. Drinking rBGH milk would thus be expected to significantly increase IGF-1 blood levels and consequently to increase risks of developing breast cancer and promoting its invasiveness.

Faced with escalating rates of breast, besides colon and prostate cancers, FDA should withdraw its approval of rBGH milk, whose sale benefits only Monsanto while posing major public health risks for the entire US population. A Congressional investigation of FDA's abdication of responsibility is well overdue.

September 1, 1998

FDA ADVISORY COMMITTEE URGED TO REJECT ZENECA'S APPLICATION OF TAMOXIFEN FOR PREVENTING BREAST CANCER IN HEALTHY WOMEN AS THE DRUG IS INEFFECTIVE AND DANGEROUS

On September 2, FDA's Advisory Committee on Oncologic Drugs will review Zeneca Pharmaceutical's New Drug Application (NDA) for approval of tamoxifen "for the prevention of breast cancer in (healthy) women at high risk." Claims that tamoxifen can prevent breast cancer are based on an April 6, 1998 National Cancer Institute (NCI) preliminary report, unsupported by a scientific publication, of a short term trial on some 13,000 healthy women at "high risk" of breast cancer, including women over the age of 60, who were randomly given tamoxifen or a placebo; further details of the report are still not available to the scientific community and the public. The trial was terminated prematurely in view of the reduction in the incidence of breast cancer in all tamoxifen treated age groups. However, serious and sometimes fatal complications, including uterine cancer and pulmonary embolism, were seen in postmenopausal women among whom the incidence of breast cancer was reduced by 1.7%, while the incidence of serious complications was increased by 2.2% in non-hysterectomized women.

The brevity of the trial prevented recognition of other delayed serious health risks. Of particular concern is the fact that tamoxifen is a highly potent carcinogen, inducing liver cancer in rats at low doses equivalent, based on blood levels, to those used in the trial. Disturbingly, women in the trial were not informed of the clear evidence of these risks. The absence of reported liver cancer in women treated with tamoxifen for breast cancer is hardly reassuring as relatively few women have been treated for over 5 years and followed up for a further 20 years before which the development of liver cancer would be most unlikely. Additionally, there are serious questions as to whether tamoxifen actually reduced the incidence of breast cancer or merely delayed its onset by treating small undetected tumors. In fact, two articles published on July 11, 1998 in the highly prestigious journal, *The Lancet*, reported no evidence of breast cancer prevention by tamoxifen in two major European trials.

In an August 17 written statement, which will be read into the record at the September 2 Advisory Committee Hearing, I concluded: "NCI's preliminary April 6 report on the prevention of breast cancer by tamoxifen has still not yet been finalized and published in a scientific journal. The Advisory Committee should also consider the propriety of Zeneca's NDA as it is based, in part, on data which have not been made fully available to the public although the underlying (NCI) research was funded by the public. Furthermore, the claimed evidence for chemoprevention has been discredited by two subsequent scientific publications. Of as great concern is the well documented evidence of short term life-threatening complications, and also risks of delayed fatal complications, evidence for which has been trivialized and suppressed by NCI. Based on these scientific and ethical considerations, the Advisory Committee is urged to deny approval of Zeneca's NDA."

Finally, the NDA poses further serious questions in view of Zeneca's control and funding of the heavily promoted annual October National

Breast Cancer Awareness Month. This campaign urges women to have mammography, in spite of its highly questionable effectiveness and risks in premenopausal women, while avoiding any reference to a wide range of scientifically documented safe and effective methods for reducing risks of breast cancer. These include avoidance of prolonged and early onset use of oral contraceptives; obesity and inactivity; and high fat and dairy food products contaminated with carcinogenic and estrogenic industrial chemicals. Such critical omissions are favorable to Zeneca's efforts to influence public policy in favor of approval of large scale tamoxifen chemoprevention, targeted for up to 30 million US women at "high risk" of breast cancer.

ENDORSERS:
Barbara Seaman
Co-Founder
National Women's Health Network
Washington, D.C.

Ann Fonfa
Annie Appleseed Project
New York

January 27, 1999

MISLEADING CLAIMS BY AN INDUSTRY-SPONSORED STUDY ON THE SAFETY OF THE PILL

A January 1999 study, funded by major international pharmaceutical companies, claims that oral contraceptives pose no risks of breast cancer or other ill effects. While the study was alleged to be the largest ever conducted, it was both small scale and insensitive. The study was based on only 23,000 healthy women who had "never used" the pill since 1968 and who were subsequently followed up over a 25 year period. The average age of women at termination of the study was only 49, an age when breast cancer is relatively uncommon. Not surprisingly, the authors admitted that the number of breast and other cancers was so small that "further data is needed to confirm our findings".

In contrast, a 1996 large scale international collaborative analysis of some 54 epidemiological studies, based on over 53,000 women with breast cancer and published in *The Lancet* in1996, demonstrated that use of the pill starting in adolescence increased risks of breast cancer by 60 percent. These risks are clearly underestimates as reflected by the authors' recognition that "there is little information about use that ceased more than 20 years ago," a latency much too short to preclude further major increases in breast cancer rates. Reliance on studies based on such short latencies would have exculpated the carcinogenicity of asbestos, besides the majority of other recognized human carcinogens. Other better designed and well controlled studies have reported much higher risks of breast cancer for women starting use of the pill in their teens or early twenties, especially with use before a full term pregnancy and subsequent prolonged use, and among women with a family history of breast cancer.

Moreover, the claim that the current low-dose synthetic ethinyl estradiol pill is much safer than the high-dose mestranol pill used in the 1960s and 1970s is misleading as the former is more potent than the latter, besides being some fortyfold more potent than natural estradiol; additionally, ethinyl estradiol, unlike mestranol, binds to estrogen receptors in the breast. Furthermore, the modern pill is used for much longer periods, often from menarche to menopause, than was the case with the earlier high-dose pills. It should further be emphasized that no studies have yet been conducted on the high potency modern pills and none are reportedly in progress. This is in striking contrast to the intensive investigation by Federal regulatory and health agencies on the endocrine-disruptive effects of estrogenic pesticides and other industrial contaminants whose potency is some 1/500,000th that of ethinyl estradiol.

Of related interest, it should be noted that the incidence of estrogen-dependent breast cancers, particularly among post-menopausal women, has increased by 130 percent from the mid-70s in sharp contrast to only a 27 percent increase in non-estrogen dependent cancers. This may well be relevant to the risks of the pill as a major source of incremental estrogen exposure.

Clearly, unqualified claims on the safety of the current pill reflect interests of the pharmaceutical industry rather than scientifically well-based concerns on women's health.

March 7, 1999

HUMAN GROWTH HORMONE ANTI-AGING
MEDICATION POSES UNDISCLOSED CANCER RISKS

Use of the genetically engineered human growth hormone (HGH) for anti-aging medication has become a major growth industry. Suppliers of HGH, including those offering mail order prescriptions, are proliferating on websites and the Internet. The Chicago-based seven-year-old American Academy of Anti-Aging Medicine, with over 8,000 members, promotes injectable HGH in programs claiming to stop or even reverse aging, including decreasing body fat, and increasing muscle mass and bone density. However, practitioners of this burgeoning "health" industry are either ignorant of or suppress well-documented information on the grave cancer risks of HGH medication.

HGH induces growth promoting and other effects by stimulating the liver to increase production of the natural Insulin-like Growth Factor-1 (IGF-1) whose blood levels normally decline with advancing age. However, there are numerous publications in prestigious peer reviewed scientific journals showing that elevated IGF-1 levels are strongly associated with major excess risks of colon, prostate, and breast cancers; even minor elevations are associated with up to 7-fold increased risks of breast cancer, risks almost as high as those in women carrying genes (BRCA1 and BRCA2) with the strongest hereditary predisposition. Additionally, IGF-1 inhibits the programmed self-destruction (apoptosis) of cancer cells, thus stimulating the growth and invasiveness of small, undiagnosed cancers, besides increasing the resistance of cancers to chemotherapy. For these reasons, anti-aging HGH medication, compounded by failure to explicitly disclose its grave risks, constitutes medical malpractice.

There are also growing concerns on possible risks from the use of HGH nutritional supplements, including oral sprays. It should, however, be recognized that HGH absorption from the mouth and gut is unlikely to be significant, in striking contrast to complete absorption from injectable medication. Nevertheless, nutritional HGH supplements should be phased out until it can be shown that they do not elevate blood IGF-1 levels.

HGH medication should only be used by qualified endocrinologists for highly restricted medical disorders, such as dwarfism due to pituitary gland deficiency, as approved by the FDA in 1985; anti-aging medication has never received such approval.

May 3, 2001

THE NATIONAL BREAST CANCER COALITION (NBCC) IS URGED BY DR. EPSTEIN TO CONSIDER BREAST EXAMINATION AS A PRACTICAL ALTERNATIVE TO MAMMOGRAPHY

The NBCC's recommendations against premenopausal mammography will be confirmed and extended by leading epidemiologists at its tenth anniversary May 5-9 Washington, D.C. meeting. However, consideration should also be given to promoting the role of breast self examination (BSE) as an effective and safe alternative to screening.

Dr. Anthony Miller, co-investigator of the recent Canadian National Breast Cancer Screening Study, will report on a unique trial of some 39,000 postmenopausal women. Half performed monthly BSE following instruction by trained nurses, had annual clinical breast examinations (CBE) by trained professionals, and also had annual mammograms. The other half practiced BSE and had annual CBE's but no mammograms. It should be noted that CBE performance by trained nurses is as good, if not better, than the study suggests. Dr. Miller concluded: "The addition of annual mammography to physical examination has no impact on breast cancer mortality". Thus, mammographic detection of non-palpable cancers failed to improve survival rates.

Dr. Peter Gotzsche, a well-known Swedish expert, further challenged claims that screening reduces breast cancer mortality by enabling early detection and treatment. Based on recent analysis of two large Swedish trials, he concluded: "There is no reliable evidence that screening decreases breast cancer mortality—(and thus that) screening is unjustified."

As detailed in a review, in press in the *International Journal of Health Services*, by Dr. Samuel Epstein, Dr. Rosalie Bertell, and Barbara Seaman, reservations on the efficacy, besides hazards, of screening are further stressed by the following considerations:

- Mammography is not a technique for early diagnosis of breast cancer which is rarely detectable until about eight years old. Screening should thus be recognized as damage control rather than, misleadingly, as "secondary prevention."

- Missed cancers are common in premenopausal women due to their dense breast structure, and also in postmenopausal women on estrogen replacement therapy who often develop breast densities, making their mammograms difficult to read. Also, about one third of all cancers, and more of the aggressive premenopausal cancers, are diagnosed between annual screenings. Women can thus be lulled into a false sense of security by an apparently negative mammogram.

- Misdiagnosed cancers are common in premenopausal women, postmenopausal women on estrogen replacement therapy, and women with a strong family history, and can reach 100% over a decade's screening. Misdiagnoses thus result in anxiety, more mammograms, unnecessary biopsies and even mastectomies.

- Over-diagnosis with subsequent overtreatment are among the major risks of mammography. With increased screening, pre-invasive breast duct cancer or ductal carcinoma-in-situ (DCIS), is now diagnosed in some 40,000 women annually and unnecessarily treated as invasive cancer by lumpectomy plus radiation or even mastectomy. However, most DCIS never becomes invasive even if untreated, and mortality is low, 1%, whether diagnosed and treated early or late.

- Screening poses cumulative cancer risks. Contrary to assurances that radiation exposure is trivial, the routine of taking four breast films results in 1 rad (radiation absorbed dose) exposure, in contrast to about one thousandth less for a chest x-ray. The premenopausal breast is highly sensitive to radiation, each rad exposure increasing cancer risk by 1%, resulting in a cumulative 10% increased risk over 10 years screening; risks are greater for "baseline" screening at younger ages. Risks are even higher for silent carriers of the A-T gene, accounting for up to 20% of all cancers. Less recognized dangers are due to the often painful breast compression during premenopausal mammography. This may rupture blood vessels in or around small undetected cancers with resulting lethal spread of malignant cells.

- Concerns on the unreliability, besides dangers, of premenopausal screening are so pervasive that this practice remains unique to the US
- Screening poses an inflationary threat; average Medicare and insurance costs are $70 and $125, respectively. If all 20 million premenopausal women had annual mammograms, minimal costs would be $2.5 billion. These costs would be quadrupled if the industry succeeds in replacing film machines, costing about $100,000, by digital machines, costing about $400,000, for which there is no evidence of improved effectiveness.

Breast examination, CBE combined with BSE, is effective, safe and low in cost in striking contrast with mammography. The American Cancer Society (ACS) admitted in 1985 that "at least 90% of the women who develop breast carcinoma discover the tumor themselves." Nevertheless, the ACS, National Cancer Institute, American College of Radiology, and the mammography industry, all remain dismissive of breast examination. Claims for the benefits of mammography screening at all ages, in a non-peer reviewed ACS publication in the May issue of Cancer, are highly flawed including by "before-after" comparisons of women unstratified by menopausal status.

National networks of CBE and BSE clinics staffed by trained nurses should be established. These clinics could further empower women by them with scientific information on breast cancer prevention of which women still remain largely unaware.

February 6, 2002

MAMMOGRAPHY IS DANGEROUS BESIDES INEFFECTIVE

Recent confirmation by Danish researchers of longstanding evidence on the ineffectiveness of screening mammography has been greeted by extensive nationwide headlines. Entirely missing from this coverage, however, has been any reference to the well-documented dangers of mammography.

Screening mammography poses significant and cumulative risks of breast cancer for premenopausal women. The routine practice of taking four films of each breast annually results in approximately 1 rad (radiation absorbed dose) exposure, about 1,000 times greater than that from a chest x-ray. The premenopausal breast is highly sensitive to radiation, each 1 rad exposure increasing breast cancer risk by about 1 percent, with a cumulative 10 percent increased risk for each breast over a decade's screening. These risks are even greater for younger women subject to "baseline screening."

Radiation risks are some four-fold greater for the 1 to 2 percent of women who are silent carriers of the A-T (ataxia-telangiectasia) gene; by some estimates this accounts for up to 20 percent of all breast cancers diagnosed annually.

Since 1928, physicians have been warned to handle "cancerous breasts with care — for fear of accidentally disseminating cells" and spreading the cancer. Nevertheless, mammography entails tight and often painful breast compression, particularly in premenopausal women, which could lead to distant and lethal spread of malignant cells by rupturing small blood vessels in or around small undetected breast cancers.

Missed cancers are common in premenopausal women owing to their dense breasts, and also in postmenopausal women on estrogen replacement therapy.

Mistakenly diagnosed cancers are common. For women with multiple risk factors including a strong family history and early menarche—just those strongly urged to have annual mammograms—the cumulative risks of false positives can reach as high as 100 percent over a decade's screening.

The widespread acceptance of screening has lead to over diagnosis of pre-invasive cancer (ductal carcinoma in situ), sometimes treated radically by mastectomy and radiation, and even chemotherapy.

As increasing numbers of premenopausal women are responding to aggressively promoted screening, imaging centers are becoming flooded. Resultantly, patients referred for diagnostic mammography are now experiencing potentially dangerous delays, up to several months, before they can be examined.

The dangers and unreliability of screening are compounded by its growing and inflationary costs. Screening all premenopausal women would cost $2.5 billion annually, about 14 percent of estimated Medicare spending on prescription drugs. These costs would be increased some fourfold if the highly profitable industry, enthusiastically supported by radiologists, succeeds in replacing film machines, costing about $100,000 each, with the latest high-tech digital machines recently approved by the FDA, costing about $400,000 each, for which there is no evidence of improved effectiveness.

The ineffectiveness and dangers of mammography pose an agonizing dilemma for the millions of women anxious for reassurance of early detection of breast cancer. However, the dilemma is more apparent than real. As proven by a September 2000 publication, based on a unique large-scale screening study by University of Toronto epidemiologists, monthly breast self-examination (BSE) following brief training, coupled with annual clinical breast examination (CBE) by a trained health care professional, is at least as effective as mammography in detecting early tumors, and also safe. National networks of BSE and CBE clinics staffed by trained nurses should be established to replace screening mammography. Apart from their minimal costs, such clinics would empower women and free them from increasing dependence on industrialized medicine and its complicit medical institutions.

May 19, 2003

GENETICALLY-ENGINEERED ANTI-AGING MEDICATION, MONSANTO MILK ARE MAJOR, UNRECOGNIZED RISKS OF BREAST CANCER

Anti-aging medication with genetically-engineered human growth hormone (HGH) poses major risks of breast cancer. Equally unrecognized are risks of drinking unlabeled milk from cows injected with Monsanto's genetically-engineered bovine growth hormone (BGH), marketed since 1994 to increase milk production. These risks are especially critical in view of the escalating incidence of breast cancer, particularly in post-menopausal women, over recent decades. As critical is the fact that women have still not been warned of both these avoidable risks.

The anti-aging effects of HGH are due to its stimulating the liver to increase production of the natural Insulin-like Growth Factor-1 (IGF-1), whose blood levels normally decline with increasing age. BGH milk also has high levels of IGF-1, which is readily absorbed through the gut.

There are numerous publications, in prestigious scientific journals since the early 1990's, showing that elevated IGF-1 levels are strongly associated with major excesses of breast, besides colon and prostate, cancer. By 1992, a leading authority on IGF-1 warned that it was strongly incriminated in the transformation of normal breast cells to cancer cells. Even minor elevations of IGF-1 are associated with up to a sevenfold increased risk of breast cancer. This is almost as high as that in women carrying genes (BRCA1 and BRCA2) with the strongest hereditary predisposition. Additionally, IGF-1 inhibits the naturally programmed ability of cancer cells to self-destruct. This results in stimulating the growth and invasiveness of small, undiagnosed cancers, and increasing their resistance to chemotherapy. These concerns on risks of high levels of IGF-1 in BGH milk are particularly strong in view of evidence that prenatal and infant breasts are highly susceptible to stimulatory and hormonal influences. This early life "imprinting" is thus likely to result in progressive increases in risks of breast cancer over future decades.

Use of HGH for anti-aging medication has become a major growth industry. Suppliers of HGH, including those offering mail order prescriptions, are proliferating on Internet web sites. The Chicago-based ten-year old American Academy of Anti-Aging Medicine, with over 8,000 members, promotes injectable HGH in programs claiming to stop or even reverse aging, including decreasing body fat, and increasing muscle mass and bone density. However, practitioners of this burgeoning "health" industry are either ignorant of or fail to warn of well-documented information on the grave cancer risks of HGH medication.

HGH medication should only be used by qualified endocrinologists for highly restricted medical disorders, such as dwarfism due to pituitary gland deficiency, as approved by the FDA in 1985. It should be further stressed that anti-aging medication has never received any such approval.

The public should also boycott unlabeled dairy products in favor of those labeled as rBGH-free, which are becoming increasingly available.

May 23, 2003

THE AMERICAN CANCER SOCIETY MISLEADS THE PUBLIC

In a one-hour special on the "TOP CANCER MYTHS," the American Cancer Society (ACS) claims to set the record straight. However, these claims are seriously flawed.

While admitting that number of people diagnosed with cancer is increasing, the ACS explains this away as due to aging of the population, and the frequency of cancer in the elderly. However, federal statistics adjusted for aging show a 24% increased incidence rate over the last three decades. What's more, most major increases have involved non-smoking related cancers. These cancers include: non-Hodgkin's lymphoma, 87%; thyroid, 71%; testis, 67%; post-menopausal breast, 54%; and brain, 28%. More disturbing is the escalating incidence of childhood cancers: acute lymphocytic leukemia, 62%; brain, 50%; bone, 40%; and kidney, 14%. Of related interest is an analysis of leading causes of death from 1973 to 1999. Cancer has increased by 30%, while mortality from heart disease decreased by 21%.

Worse still, the ACS has failed to inform the public about scientifically well-documented causes of a wide range of non-smoking related cancers. The ACS goes further by dismissing evidence on risks from domestic use of pesticides, although several studies have clearly shown a strong relationship with childhood cancers. In its recommendation for high vegetable, fruit, and grain diets, ACS ignores the fact that these, including baby foods, are highly contaminated with carcinogenic pesticides, while ignoring the availability of safe organic products. The ACS goes even further in dismissing such concerns. In its Cancer Facts and Figures 2002, ACS reassured that cancer risks from dietary pesticides, besides hazardous waste sites, and ionizing radiation from "closely controlled" nuclear plants, are at such low levels as to be "negligible."

The CANCER MYTHS are consistent with its longstanding track record on prevention, policies, and conflicts of interest. In 1978, the ACS refused a Congressional request to support the Clean Air Act. In 1992, the ACS supported the Chlorine Institute by defending the continued use of carcinogenic chlorinated pesticides. In 1993, just before PBS aired the Frontline special, "In Our Children's Food," the ACS came out in support of the pesticide industry. In a damage- control memorandum, sent to some 48 regional divisions and their 3,000 local offices, the ACS trivialized pesticides as a cause of childhood cancer. ACS also reassured the public that food contaminated with carcinogenic pesticides is safe, even for babies.

In 1994, the ACS published a highly flawed study designed to reassure women on the safety of dark permanent hair dyes, and to trivialize the risks of non-Hodgkin's lymphoma, breast, and other cancers as documented in over six prior reports.

Analysis of the 1998 ACS budget revealed that it allocated less than 0.1% of its $700 million revenues to "Environmental Carcinogenesis."

In 2000, it was discovered that the ACS had close ties to PR firms for the tobacco industry—Shandwick International, representing R.J. Reynolds Holdings, and Edelman, representing Brown & Williamson Tobacco Company. These firms were promptly dismissed once the embarrassing news leaked out.

This indifference or hostility of the ACS to cancer prevention is less surprising in view of its pervasive conflicts of interest with the cancer drug, petrochemical, cosmetics, power plants, and other industries.

Not surprisingly, the authoritative US charity watchdog, The Chronicle of Philanthropy, has warned against the transfer of money from the public purse to private hands. "The ACS is more interested in accumulating wealth than in saving lives."

For a detailed critique of the ACS track record and policies, see the Cancer Prevention Coalition February 2003 "Stop Cancer Before It Starts Campaign" report at http://www.preventcancer.com/; the report has been endorsed by some 100 leading experts in cancer prevention, and representatives of consumer, environmental, and activist groups.

November 4, 2003
AN OUNCE OF PREVENTION

Cancer has become the leading cause of disease and death in the United States. A much higher priority for prevention would reduce this carnage, and the need for treatment.

In 1971, Congress passed the National Cancer Act and Program. This was prompted by well orchestrated appeals from leading representatives of the "cancer establishment," the federal National Cancer Institute (NCI) and the world's wealthiest nonprofit organization, the American Cancer Society (ACS). They promised that the cure for cancer was imminent, but only if given an increase in NCI's funding.

Spurred on by a major media campaign, aggressively promoted by NCI and ACS representatives, including a full page advertisement in the *New York Times*, "Mr. Nixon, You Can Cure Cancer," President Richard Nixon enthusiastically embraced the Act. He launched the "War Against Cancer," increased NCI's 1971 budget from $150 to $220 million, and gave NCI unprecedented autonomy.

Unfortunately, the Act had unintended consequences. The Act authorized the President to appoint the director of the NCI, and authorize its budget, thus bypassing the director of all the other 26 National Institutes of Health. The Act thus effectively insulated and politicized the National Cancer Institute.

Over 30 years and some $55 billion later, we are further away from winning the cancer war than when it was first declared. But that is contrary to what we had been led to believe.

Since passage of the 1971 Act, the National Cancer Institute and the ACS have reassured the nation with a steady stream of misleading press releases, briefings, and media reports hailing major progress in the cancer war.

These include repeated claims for miracle "breakthroughs" in cancer treatment, and also the 1984 and 1986 NCI promises that cancer mortality would be halved by 2000.

The misleading statements include the 1998 reassurances by the NCI and ACS that the nation had "turned the corner" in the war on cancer, and the February 11, 2003 incredible "pledge" by NCI director Dr. Andrew von Eschenbach to "eliminate the suffering and death from cancer by 2015."

Also misleading is the September 2003 claim, in the "Annual Report to the Nation on the Status of Cancer, 1975-2000," by the NCI, co-authored by the ACS, and the Centers for Disease Control and Prevention, that "considerable progress has been made in reducing the burden of cancer."

These claims don't even pass the laugh test. Cancer mortality rates have remained virtually unchanged (199/100,000) from 1975 to 2000. These rates are based on NCI's statistics, which are adjusted to compensate for the aging population.

Over the same period, overall cancer incidence rates have escalated by 18 percent, now striking about 1.3 million annually. Today, nearly one in two men and more than one in three women develop cancer in their lifetimes.

This translates into approximately 56 percent more cancer in men, and 22 percent more cancer in women over the course of a single generation. Cancer has become a disease of "mass destruction."

Contrary to what one might think, this increase is not due to smoking. Lung cancer rates have dropped sharply due to decreased smoking by men over recent decades.

Furthermore, the increased incidence rates from 1975 to 2000 involve many cancers unrelated to smoking. These include: non-Hodgkin's lymphoma (71 percent); testes (54 percent); thyroid (54 percent); breast (29 percent); and acute myeloid leukemia (15 percent). For African Americans, cancer rates are even higher, with excesses up to 120 percent.

Childhood cancers now strike about 9,000 young people each year and are killing about 1,500 annually. From 1975 to 2000, childhood cancer rates have increased dramatically. These include: acute lymphocytic leukemia (59 percent), brain cancer (48 percent), kidney cancer (43 percent), and bone cancer (20 percent).

The escalating incidence of childhood and non-smoking related adult cancers is paralleled by NCI's escalating budget from $220 million in 1971 to the current $4.6 billion, a 30-fold increase.

Paradoxically, it seems that the more we spend on cancer, the more cancer we get.

The reason why we are losing the winnable cancer war is because the cancer establishment's priorities remain fixated on damage control—screening, diagnosis, and treatment—and related basic research.

All these are unarguably important, and deserve substantial funding. However, much less funding would be needed if more cancer was prevented, with less cancer to treat.

The pro-industry agenda of the American Cancer Society is exemplified by its minuscule prevention research budget. In spite of bloated contrary claims, less than 0.1 percent of its $800 million budget has been allocated to research on the prevention of environmental carcinogenesis.

ACS' financial ties to the cancer drug and polluting industries remain extensive. Over 25 drug and biotech companies are Excalibur donors, who each have contributed in excess of $100,000 annually. These include: Bristol-Myers Squibb, Pfizer, AstraZeneca, Eli Lilly, Amgen, Genentech, and Johnson & Johnson.

Polluting industries that are donors include over 10 petrochemical and oil companies, such as British Petroleum, DuPont, Akzo Nobel, Pennzoil and Concho Oil. Other donors include global cosmetic companies, such as Elizabeth Arden, Revlon, Christian Dior, and Givaudan.

A total of some 300 other industries and companies make similar contributions to ACS's $800 million annual budget, a figure that excludes government grants, and income from about $1 billion in reserves. These figures hardly justify annual appeals, claiming the need for more funds to continue support of ongoing cancer programs.

As might be anticipated, the ACS returns its donors' favors with more than a wink and a nod. The society has supported the automobile industry in refusing to endorse the Clean Air Act. It has joined the Chlorine Institute in defending the continued manufacture of chlorinated carcinogenic pesticides. And it has supported the cosmetic industry in failing to warn women of risks of breast and other cancers from permanent black hair dyes, and of risks of ovarian cancer from sanitary dusting with talc.

Not surprisingly, "The Chronicle of Philanthropy," the nation's leading charity watchdog, charged in 1992 that, "The ACS is more interested in accumulating wealth than saving lives." The Chronicle also warned against the transfer of money from the public purse to private hands.

The most disturbing development in the cancer war has been its privatization by the ACS. In 1998, the ACS created and funded the National Dialogue on Cancer (NDC), co-chaired by former President George Bush, and Barbara Bush. Included were a wide range of cancer survivor groups, some 100 representatives of the cancer drug industry, and Shandwick International PR, whose major clients include R.J. Reynolds Tobacco Holdings.

In the "Cancer Letter," an insider cancer publication which has investigated the NDC from its onset, Dr. Durant charged the ACS with "protecting their own fund raising capacity ... from competition by survivor groups. It has always seemed to me that this was an issue of control by the ACS over the cancer agenda."

Without informing NDC's participants, and behind closed doors, the American Cancer Society then spun off a small Legislative Committee. Its explicit objective was to advise Congress on the need to replace the 1971 National Cancer Act with a new National Cancer Control Act. The new Act is intended to shift major control of cancer policy from the public National Cancer Institute to the nonprofit American Cancer Society.

The proposed Act would also increase NCI funding from this year's $4.6 billion to $14 billion by 2007. The American Cancer Society was assisted by Shandwick in drafting the new Act and managing the National Dialogue on Cancer.

Following the embarrassing January 2000 disclosure that R.J. Reynolds Tobacco Holdings was one of Shandwick's major clients, about which the ACS claimed it has been unaware, the PR firm was promptly fired.

But then, ACS hired another well known tobacco PR firm, Edelman Public Relations Worldwide, to conduct a voter cancer education campaign for the 2000 Presidential elections.

Edelman represents the Brown & Williamson Tobacco Company, and The Altria Group, the parent company of Philip Morris, the nation's biggest cigarette maker.

With the February 2002 appointment of ACS President-Elect von Eschenbach as National Cancer Institute director, the National Cancer Program was effectively privatized.

Commenting on the ACS relationship with the tobacco industry, prominent anti-smoking activist Dr. Stanton Glantz said, "It's like ... Bush hiring Al Qaeda to do PR, because they have good connections to Al-Jazeera."

Playing the other side of the coin, on August 19 the ACS announced strong support for increasing the Food and Drug Administration's authority to regulate tobacco products.

Meanwhile, the good cop/bad cop relationship between the ACS and the tobacco industry and other polluting industries continues to escape public attention.

As disturbing is the growing secretive collaboration between the NCI and the ACS-NDC complex, as revealed in the August 2003 Cancer Letter.

The latest example is the joint planning of a massive tumor tissue bank. This would cost between $500 million and $1.2 billion to operate, apart from construction costs in the billions.

This initiative would be privatized, rife with conflicts of interest, exempt from the provisions of the Federal Advisory Committee and Freedom of Information Acts, and free from federal technology transfer regulations.

These developments, coupled with the NCI's track record on prevention, fully justify the recommendations of the July 2003 report by The National Academy of Sciences (NAS).

The report stressed the autonomous "special status" of the NCI, resulting in "an unnecessary rift between (its) goals and leadership" and those of the National Institutes of Health.

More seriously, control of the nation's cancer agenda has been surreptitiously transferred from the public to the private sector's special interests.

A Congressional investigation of these critical concerns, and NCI's failure to implement the National Cancer Act's mandate is decades overdue.

ENDORSER:
Quentin D. Young, M.D.
Chairman of the Health and Medicine Policy Research Group
Past President of the American Public Health Association

October 28, 2005

THE LOOK GOOD . . . FEEL BETTER PROGRAM: BUT AT WHAT RISK?

Launched in 1989 by the Cosmetic, Toiletry, and Fragrance Association (CTFA) and the National Cosmetology Association, the Look Good . . . Feel Better Program is "dedicated to teaching women cancer patients beauty techniques to help restore their appearance and self-image during cancer treatment." About 30,000 breast and other cancer patients participate yearly, each receiving a free makeover and bag of makeup.

Just what could be more noble? Or so it might just seem. The Look Good Program is supported by 22 CTFA-member cosmetic companies, including multibillion-dollar household name global giants. Each year, member companies "donate over one million individual cosmetic and personal care products, valued at $10 million, and raise more than $2 million." The Program is administered nationwide by the American Cancer Society (ACS), "which manages volunteer training, and serves as the primary source of information to the public."

There is no doubt that the products donated by the cosmetic companies, such as eye and cheek colors, lipsticks, moisture lotions, pressed powders and other makeup, are restorative. However, there is also no doubt that the ACS and the companies involved are oblivious to or strangely silent on the dangers of the Look Good products, whose ingredients are readily absorbed through the skin.

A review of 12 Look Good products, marketed by six companies, reveals that 10 contain dangerous chemical ingredients. Based on longstanding scientific evidence, these pose risks of cancer, and also hormonal (endocrine disruptive) effects.

Evidence for the cancer risks is based on standard tests in rodents, and on human (epidemiological) studies. Evidence for the hormonal risks is based on test-tube tests with breast cancer cells, or by stimulating premature sexual development in infant rodents. Unbelievably, the ACS explicitly warns women undergoing chemotherapy—"Don't use hormonal creams."

Take for example Estee Lauder's LightSource Transforming Moisture Lotion, Chanel's Sheer Lipstick, and Merle Norman Eye Color. These products contain ingredients which are carcinogenic, contaminated with carcinogens, or precursors of carcinogens. The products also contain hormonal ingredients, known as parabens, one of which has been identified in breast cancer tissue, and incriminated as a probable cause of breast cancer.

The ACS silence with regard to the risks of the Look Good products extends more widely to cosmetics and personal care products used by women, personal care products used by men, and baby lotions and shampoos. This silence is also consistent with the imbalanced objectives of the ACS highly publicized annual "Breast Cancer Awareness Month." While dedicated to the early detection of breast cancer, this event is silent on a wide range of its avoidable causes, besides the escalating incidence of post-menopausal breast cancer, by nearly 40%, over the last three decades.

Of likely relevance to the ACS silence is its interlocking interests with the cosmetic, besides other industries. The major Look Good companies are among some 350 ACS "Excalibur Donors," each donating a minimum of $10,000 annually. Other donors include petrochemical, power plant, and hazardous waste industries, whose environmental pollutants have been incriminated as causes of breast, besides other, cancers. Not surprisingly, The Chronicle of Philanthropy, the nation's leading charity watchdog, has charged that "The ACS is more interested in accumulating wealth than saving lives."

The ACS silence is also shared by the National Cancer Institute (NCI), which is required by the 1971 National Cancer Act to provide the public with information on avoidable causes of cancer. In spite of $50 billion tax-payers funding since 1971, the NCI has joined with the ACS in denying the public's right to know of avoidable causes of cancer from industrial chemicals, radiation, and common prescription drugs. Both the NCI and ACS are locked at the hip in policies fixated on damage control-screening, diagnosis, treatment and treatment-related research-with indifference to cancer prevention due to avoidable exposures to chemical carcinogens in cosmetics, other consumer products, air and water.

Equally asleep at the wheel remains the Food and Drug Administration in spite of its explicit regulatory authority. The 1938 Federal Food, Drug and Cosmetic Act explicitly requires that "The label of cosmetic products shall bear a warning statement . . . to prevent a health hazard that may be associated with a product."

No wonder the nation is losing the winnable war against cancer.

June 27, 2006

HORMONAL MILK POSES GREATER RISKS THAN JUST TWINNING

As widely covered in the national media, a recent article by Dr. Gary Steinman in the *Journal of Reproductive Medicine* reported that women drinking milk and eating dairy products from cows injected with Monsanto's genetically engineered growth hormone drug are up to five times more likely to risk giving birth to fraternal twins than non-dairy product vegans.

This news is hardly surprising. Hormonal milk contains up to ten-fold increased levels of the natural Insulin-like Growth Factor, known as IGF, long known to increase ovulation and twinning rates in cows. The hormone also makes cows sick. Monsanto has been forced to admit to 20 toxic veterinary effects on its drug label.

Monsanto has also recently admitted that about one third of dairy cows in the nation are now in herds where the hormone is used.

Hormonal milk is very different than natural milk. Hormonal milk is often contaminated with pus cells, resulting from mastitis in cows due to hyperstimulation of milk production, and also with antibiotics used to treat the mastitis. Other abnormalities include increased fatty acids, which are incriminated in heart disease.

More serious are major risks of breast, colon, and prostate cancers due to increased IGF levels in hormonal milk. Evidence for this has been documented in about 50 scientific publications over the past three decades. Among them is the 1998 Harvard Nurses Health Study, based on a follow-up of 300 healthy nurses. Those with elevated IGF blood levels were shown to have up to a seven-fold increased risk of breast cancer.

A less well-recognized risk is evidence that IGF blocks natural, self-destructive, defense mechanisms against early submicroscopic cancers, technically known as apoptosis.

Acting on these lines of evidence, a 1999 European Commission Report, by internationally recognized experts, concluded that avoidance of hormonal dairy products in favor of natural organic products "would appear to be the most practical and immediate dietary intervention to . . . achieve the goal of preventing cancer." Warning of these risks were confirmed in my 2002 publication in the *International Journal of Health Services*, endorsed by over 50 leading independent experts in cancer prevention and public health.

Of particular concern are risks to infants and children in view of their high susceptibility to cancer-causing products and chemicals. Nevertheless, few schools make organic milk available, nor do most state governments, under low-income food programs, particularly the Special Supplemental Nutrition Program for Women, Infants and Children.

Nevertheless, the Food and Drug Administration remains indifferent to these risks, in spite of Congressional concerns. Illustrative is the 1986 report, "Human Food Safety and Regulation of Animal Drugs," by the House Committee on Government Operations. This concluded that the "FDA has consistently disregarded its responsibility—has repeatedly put what it perceives are interests of veterinarians and the livestock industry ahead of its legal obligations to protect consumers—jeopardizing the health and safety of consumers of meat, milk, and poultry."

However, these risks are avoidable. According to The Hartman Group, a prominent Seattle consulting firm, organic milk is now among the first organic product that consumers buy. Organic milk is also becoming increasingly available, with an annual growth rate of about 20 percent, while overall milk consumption is dropping by about 10 percent.

Wal-Mart is now the biggest seller of certified organic milk, followed by Horizon Organic, owned by Dean Foods, the nation's largest dairy producer, and by Groupe Danone, the leading French dairy company. While growth in this market is still held back by the higher price of organic milk, this problem is likely to be resolved by Wal-Mart's competitive pricing.

In sharp contrast to the US, 24 European nations, Norway, Switzerland, New Zealand, Japan, and Canada have banned the use and imports of hormonal milk and dairy products. However, in spite of the ban, Canada imports over 20 percent of its total dairy products from the US, without any restrictions.

Our government has failed to warn its citizens of the dangers of hormonal milk. The media could now play a critical role in alerting the nation to these avoidable dangers.

April 2, 2007

THE UNITED NATIONS TAKES THE INITIATIVE IN THE WAR AGAINST CANCER

This week, after notables such as Elizabeth Edwards and Tony Snow, have shared the bad news with the nation that their cancers have returned, we are deluged with a series of editorials in last Sunday's *New York Times*. These emphasize early screening, the latest promise of new treatment modalities, and the latest promise of new genetic research. However, not once in any of these editorials or other news items is the word prevention even mentioned.

Rather than winning the cancer war, we have been losing it progressively since President Richard Nixon declared the War on Cancer in 1971. Today, cancer strikes nearly 1.3 million people annually. Nearly one in two men and more than one in three women develop cancer in their lifetimes. This translates into approximately 56 percent more cancer in men and 22 percent more cancer in women over the course of just one generation.

Since 1971, and with some $50 billion taxpayers funding of the National Cancer Institute, the incidence of a wide range of cancers unrelated to smoking has escalated to near epidemic proportions. These include: thyroid cancer by over 80%; childhood leukemia by 70%; non-Hodgkin's lymphoma by 70%; and testes cancer by 50%.

More disturbingly, there is long-standing, well-documented epidemiological evidence on the avoidable causes of these cancers, notably environmental and occupational carcinogens. There is also well documented evidence on carcinogenic ingredients and contaminants in common consumer products-food, cosmetics and personal care products, and household products.

However, this evidence is ignored or trivialized by the National Cancer Institute in lock step with the world's largest charity, the American Cancer Society. This charity has been characterized by *The Chronicle of Philanthropy*, the nation's leading charity watchdog, as "more interested in accumulating wealth than saving lives."

Responding to these critical concerns, the United Nations has just announced a critical initiative on "Meeting the Global Challenge of Cancer." This has been created in response to the World Health Organization's warning that "We are now on the brink of an international cancer epidemic, with cancer now representing far more deaths than HIV, AIDS, tuberculosis, and malaria combined."

The United Nations has recently invited Dr. Samuel S. Epstein and Dr. Nicholas Ashford to take a lead role in launching its Stop Cancer initiative, and on how to win the losing cancer war, an invitation we have readily accepted.

ENDORSER:

Nicholas A. Ashford, PhD., JD

Professor of Technology and Policy

Director, MIT Technology and Law Program

Massachusetts Institute of Technology

May 16, 2007

AVOIDABLE CAUSES OF BREAST CANCER

The Silent Spring Institute must be warmly commended for compiling very important and well-documented reports on environmental causes of breast cancer, termed "mammary gland carcinogens."

These reports clearly incriminate a wide range of industrial chemicals which have been shown over recent decades to induce breast cancer in standard carcinogenicity tests in rats and mice.

Surprisingly, however, the reports make no reference to unarguable epidemiological evidence on other "mammary gland carcinogens," particularly FDA approved drugs; oral contraceptives; estrogen replacement therapy; and rBGH, a genetically engineered drug, injected in cows to increase milk production.

A long-standing series of studies over the last three decades have clearly incriminated hormonal contraceptives as major risks of breast cancer. These include:

- A 1981 study in the *British Journal of Cancer* reported a nearly four-fold increased risk in young women who had used oral contraceptives for eight years before their first pregnancy.

- In 1982, the *American Journal of Epidemiology* announced that women aged 35 to 54 who used oral contraceptives before their first childbirth tripled their risks of breast cancer.

- A 1987 study in the *British Journal of Cancer* reported that women under the age of 45 who had used the Pill for over four years before their first full-term pregnancy more than doubled their risk.

- A 1988 study published in *Neoplasia* reported that the risk of breast cancer increased with duration of use of the Pill, particularly for seven or more years. This risk increased to more than seven fold in women with a family history.

- In 1988, the Cancer and Steroid Hormone Study, published in *Contraception*, revealed that women who had used oral contraceptives for eight years or more, who had never given birth, and who had begun menstruating before the age of 13 were at increased risk for developing breast cancer before the age of 45. The risk was nearly three-fold for eight to eleven years of use, and twelvefold for twelve or more years of use.
- In 1995, a National Cancer Institute study found a strong link between the length of time oral contraceptives are used and breast cancer risk. A few months of use could increase a woman's risk by 30 percent. An over two-fold risk was found with ten years of use.

The evidence incriminating estrogen replacement therapy (ERT) as a major risk of breast cancer is also long standing and extensive.

- In 1991, an *American Journal of Epidemiology* article cited eight major studies demonstrating up to 80 percent increased risk of breast cancer among women using ERT for extended periods.
- In 1991, pooled results from sixteen previous studies, published in the *Journal of the American Medical Association*, found that women who used ERT for fifteen years increased their risk of breast cancer by 30 percent. Ten fold higher risks were reported among women with a family history of breast cancer.
- In 1995, the Harvard Nurses' Health Study confirmed an increased risk of 30 to 70 percent for women on ERT.
- A large-scale study, based on 60,000 postmenopausal women, published in the 1997 New England Journal of Medicine, showed that the use of ERT for over 10 years increased breast cancer deaths by 43 percent.

Also surprising is the failure of the report to make any reference to over 20 publications demonstrating up to a sevenfold increased risk of breast cancer from consumption of milk from cows injected with the genetically engineered bovine growth hormone rBGH drug, as approved by the FDA. This evidence is detailed by the author and four colleagues in a May 11, 2007 Citizen Petition to the FDA (www.preventcancer.com).

Evidence of these avoidable causes of breast cancer also lends urgent support for current Senate proposals calling for radical reform of the US Food and Drug Administration to ensure that drugs are safe as advertised.

October 16, 2007

THE BREAST CANCER AWARENESS MONTH MISLEADS WOMEN

In 1984, the American Cancer Society (ACS) inaugurated the National Breast Cancer Awareness Month (NBCAM), with its October 17 flagship National Mammography Day. The NBCAM was conceived and funded by the Imperial Chemical Industries, a leading international manufacturer of petrochemicals, and its US subsidiary Zeneca Pharmaceuticals. Zeneca is the sole manufacturer of tamoxifen, claimed to reduce risks of breast cancer, even though it is toxic and carcinogenic.

The NBCAM assured women that "early (mammography) detection results in a cure nearly 100% of the time." More specifically, the NBCAM is primarily directed to claims for reducing the incidence and mortality of breast cancer through early detection by annual mammography starting at age 40.

Still unrecognized by the ACS, and also the National Cancer Institute (NCI), is strong evidence that mammography poses significant risks of breast cancer. The routine practice of taking four films annually for each breast results in approximately 1 rad (radiation absorbed dose) exposure, which is approximately 1,000 times the dose from a single chest X-ray. Each rad exposure increases risks of breast cancer by about one percent, with a cumulative 10 percent increased risk for each breast over a decade's screening.

Moreover, the premenopausal breast is highly sensitive to radiation. Not surprisingly, premenopausal mammography screening is practiced by no nation other than the US. Risks of premenopausal mammography are some four-fold greater for the one to two percent of women who are carriers of the A-T gene (ataxia telangiectasia), and highly sensitive to the carcinogenic effects of radiation. By some estimates, this accounts for up to 20 percent of all breast cancers diagnosed annually.

Compounding these problems, missed cancers are common in premenopausal women due to the density of their breasts.

That most breast cancers are first recognized by women was admitted in 1985 by the ACS. "We must keep in mind that at least 90% of the women who develop breast cancer discover the tumors themselves." Furthermore, an analysis of several 1993 studies showed that women who regularly performed breast self-examination (BSE) detected their cancers much earlier than women failing to examine themselves. The effectiveness of BSE however depends on training by skilled professionals, enhanced by annual clinical breast examination by a professional. In spite of such evidence, the ACS and radiologists dismiss BSE, and claim that "no studies have clearly shown the benefit of using BSE."

A leading Massachusetts newspaper featured a photograph of two women in their twenties in an ACS advertisement that promised early detection by mammography results in a cure "nearly 100 percent of the time." An ACS communications director, questioned by journalist Kate Dempsey, responded in an article published in the Massachusetts Women's Community's journal *Cancer*. "The ad isn't based on a study. When you make an advertisement, you just say what you can to get women in the door. You exaggerate a point . . . Mammography today is a lucrative [and] highly competitive business." She just couldn't be any more correct.

With this background, it is not surprising that the NBCAM neglects to inform women how they can reduce their risks of breast cancer. In fact, we know a great deal about its avoidable causes which are trivialized or ignored by the ACS. These include:

- Prolonged use of the Pill or estrogen replacement therapy.
- High consumption of meat which is heavily contaminated with potent natural or synthetic estrogens, or other sex hormones, implanted in cattle in feedlots prior to slaughter to increase muscle mass.
- Prolonged consumption of milk from cows injected with a genetically engineered growth hormone to increase milk production. This milk is contaminated with high levels of a natural growth factor, which increases breast cancer risks by up to seven-fold.
- Prolonged exposure to a wide range of unlabeled hormonal ingredients in cosmetics and personal care products.
- Living near hazardous waste sites, petrochemical plants, power lines, and nuclear plants.

- Occupational exposures of over one million women to carcinogens. These include benzene, ethylene oxide, methylene chloride, phenylenediamine hair dyes, and agricultural pesticides, including DDT residues.

ENDORSER:

Rosalie Bertell, PhD

Former President of the International Institute of Concern for Public Health, Toronto, Canada

Regent of the International Physicians for Humanitarian Medicine, Geneva, Switzerland

June 15, 2009
MEDICAL EXPERTS PRESCRIBE LEGISLATION TO HELP PREVENT CANCER

A letter to Congressional leaders urging drastic revision of the Obama Cancer Plan to mandate prevention was released today by medical and scientific experts on the causes and prevention of cancer.

The letter expressing their concern that cancer prevention has received no attention in the Obama plan is addressed to four congressional committees: the Senate Committee on Health, Education, Labor and Pensions; the Senate Appropriations Committee; the House Committee on Energy and Commerce; and the House Appropriations Committee.

The experts recommend that Congress enact legislative reforms to the 1971 National Cancer Act, including a statement that it is the national policy of the United States to reduce carcinogenic exposures by at least half during the next decade. They also urge the annual publication of a comprehensive public register of carcinogens.

The scientists and doctors prescribe major policy changes for the National Cancer Institute (NCI). These include the appointment of a new Deputy Director for Cancer Prevention, and the allocation of at least 40% of the NCI budget to prevention programs for Fiscal Year 2011.

The text of the letter follows.

Dear Senators and Representatives;

President Obama has boldly pledged to reform the national health care system. Central to this, as the president has stressed, is containing the spiraling costs of health care—costs which are soaring at about 6% each year. Most experts agree that this is not possible without a better plan to prevent Americans from getting cancer in the first place. This year, 1.5 million people will be diagnosed with cancer. Of them, 562,000 people—over 1,500 every day—will die.

The cancer epidemic strikes as many as one in three Americans and takes the life of one in four. After 37 years of losing the war against cancer (a war that President Nixon originally declared in December 1971), we are taking grossly and demonstrably inadequate action to protect us from this menace.

While research on the prevention and treatment of cancer is predominantly the responsibility of the National Cancer Institute (NCI), other governmental agencies are also involved. These include the Environmental Protection Agency (EPA), the Occupational Safety and Health Administration (OSHA), the Consumer Product Safety Commission (CPSC), and the Food and Drug Administration (FDA). Unfortunately, such action is uncoordinated and unbalanced.

The connection between our losing the cancer war and the need to control costs through prevention is clear. Cancer is not only one of the most costly and sometimes deadly diseases in America, it is also one of the most preventable.

Based on recent estimates by the National Institutes of Health, the total costs of cancer are $219 billion a year. The annual costs to taxpayers of diagnosis and treatment amount to $89 billion; the annual costs of premature death are conservatively estimated at $112 billion; and the annual costs due to lost productivity are conservatively estimated at $18 billion. And these are the quantifiable, inflationary economic costs. The human costs surely are of far greater magnitude.

To be sure, smoking remains the best-known and single largest cause of cancer, particularly lung cancer. While incidence rates of lung cancer in men have declined by 20% over the past three decades, rates in women increased by 111%. But more importantly, non-smoking cancers—due to known chemical and physical carcinogens—have increased substantially since 1975. Some of the more startling realities in the failure to prevent cancer are illustrated by their soaring rates of increase. These include:

- Breast cancer is increasing 17% due to a wide range of factors. These include: birth control pills; estrogen replacement therapy; toxic hormonal ingredients in cosmetics and personal care products; diagnostic radiation; and routine premenopausal mammography, with a cumulative breast dose exposure of up to about five rads over ten years. Reflecting these concerns, Representatives Debbie Wasserman-Schultz and Henry Waxman have introduced bills promoting educational campaigns, including teaching regular breast self examination to high school students. However, and in spite of its scientifically proven efficacy, this initiative has been strongly challenged by breast cancer prevention "experts" who remain unaware of the scientific evidence on the cancer risks of high dose radiation premenopausal mammography. Furthermore, these "experts" are unaware of the well-documented scientific evidence of avoidable causes of breast cancer, other than factors related to . . . "childbirth and breastfeeding."
- Malignant melanoma of the skin in adults is increasing by 168% due to the use of sunscreens in childhood that fail to block long wave ultraviolet light;
- Thyroid cancer is increasing by 124% due in large part to ionizing radiation;
- Non-Hodgkin's lymphoma is increasing 76% due mostly to phenoxy herbicides; and phenylenediamine hair dyes;
- Testicular cancer is increasing by 49% due to pesticides; hormonal ingredients in cosmetics and personal care products; and estrogen residues in meat;
- Childhood leukemia is increasing by 55% due to ionizing radiation; domestic pesticides; nitrite preservatives in meats, particularly hot dogs; and parental exposures to occupational carcinogens;
- Ovary cancer (mortality) for women over the age of 65 has increased by 47% in African American women and 13% in Caucasian women due to genital use of talc powder.

It is now beyond dispute in the independent scientific community that environmental and occupational exposures to carcinogens are the primary cause of non-smoking related cancers. An October 2007 publication on environmental and occupational causes of cancer by one of us (Dr. Richard Clapp) further emphasized that the increasing incidence of cancer is due to preventable exposures to carcinogens in the workplace and environment.

The Clapp report provides a wide range of evidence showing preventable cancers resulting from environmental exposures to formaldehyde, chlorinated organic pesticides, and organic solvents, among other substances.

The Clapp report also cites a wealth of evidence attributing the increasing incidence of lung cancers to preventable occupational exposures to asbestos, silica, chromium VI, formaldehyde, methylene chloride, benzene, and ethylene oxide.

The National Cancer Institute is the primary federal agency devoted exclusively to fighting cancer. Paradoxically, the escalating incidence of cancer over the last thirty years parallels its sharply escalating annual budget—from $690 million in 1975 to $6 billion this year. Of this a mere $131 million is allocated to NCI's mission on Prevention and Early Detection. Furthermore, President Obama has proposed a 5% increase in funding the NCI for unspecified cancer research, with a doubling to $11.5 billion over the next eight years.

However, in spite of well-documented evidence relating the escalating incidence of cancer to a wide range of avoidable carcinogenic exposures, the NCI remains "asleep at the wheel," and has stubbornly refused to devote significant resources or even attention to prevention.

The NCI has also ignored proddings from Congress and independent scientific experts to develop a comprehensive registry of carcinogens. Worse still, the NCI has misled the public by claiming that most cancers are due to unhealthy behavior, "blaming the victim," despite overwhelming evidence to the contrary.

NCI officials still claim, for instance that 94% of all cancers are due to "unhealthy behavior" such as smoking, poor nutrition, inactivity, obesity and over exposure to sunlight—and that a mere 6% are attributable to exposures to environmental and occupational exposures.

These estimates are based on those published in 1981 by the late U.K. epidemiologist Sir Richard Doll. However, from 1976 to 1999, Doll had been a closet consultant to U.K. and US industries, including General

Motors, Monsanto and the asbestos industry. Following revelation of these conflicts of interest and just prior to his death in 2002, Doll finally admitted that most cancers, other than those related to smoking and hormones, "are induced by exposure to chemicals often environmental."

Meanwhile, the NCI has touted the imminent success of new cancer treatments—promises that have seldom borne out, and which have been widely questioned by the independent scientific community. For instance, in 2004, Nobel Laureate Leland Hartwell, President of the Fred Hutchinson Cancer Control Center, warned that Congress and the public are paying NCI $4.7 billion a year, most of which is spent on "promoting ineffective drugs" for terminal disease.

As members of the independent scientific community, we welcome the Obama Administration's goal of health care reform and prevention. But while President Obama has put forward a unique cancer plan, it focuses far too much on the diagnosis and treatment of cancer, rather than on prevention. The simple truth is that the more cancer is prevented, the less there is to treat. That will also save lives and money.

Congress now has an epochal opportunity to reform our health care system and prevent diseases, particularly cancer, from occurring in the first place. By taking some simple steps, Congress should enact reforms to prevent cancer. Accordingly, we recommend that Congress enact the following specific legislative reforms to the 1971 National Cancer Act:

- Congress declares that it is the national policy of the United States to reduce carcinogenic exposures to confirmed or suspected carcinogens by at least half during the next decade.

- Congress shall create a Deputy Director for Cancer Prevention of the NCI who, in consultation with the administrators of EPA, OSHA, CPSC, FDA and other relevant regulatory agencies, shall report to Congress annually on steps needed during the next decade, under existing regulatory authority, to reduce, by at least half, exposures reasonably anticipated to reduce the prevalence of future preventable cancers.

- The Deputy Director of NCI shall meet quarterly with the administrators of EPA, OSHA, CPSC, FDA and other relevant regulatory agencies to identify opportunities to reduce exposures to carcinogens in the environment, the workplace, pharmaceuticals, and consumer products—food, household products, and cosmetics and personal care products.

- The Deputy Director's annual report shall include recommendations for changes in statutes, regulations and enforcement authority, necessary to achieve this national policy, in consultation with the administrators of the EPA, OSHA, CPSC, FDA and other relevant regulatory agencies.
- Congress shall allocate at least 40% of the NCI budget to explicit prevention related programs for FY 2011, and 50% by FY 2014.
- Congress shall mandate the annual publication of a comprehensive register of carcinogens. This will provide federal, state and local governments, as well as the public, with comprehensive information on carcinogens in the workplace, environment, and consumer products so that necessary preventive action can be promptly undertaken.

These steps alone will not win the war against cancer, but they will be critical in redirecting a failing war on cancer that can best be described as one of the most notorious public health failures of the 20th century. Cancer prevention is a critical public policy area in which reform is long overdue.

EXPERTS ON CAUSES AND PREVENTION OF CANCER:

Nicholas A. Ashford, PhD., JD, Professor of Technology and Policy, Director, MIT Technology and Law Program, Massachusetts Institute of Technology

Richard W. Clapp, DSc, MPH, Professor Environmental Health, Boston University School of Public Health

Quentin D. Young, MD, Past President American Public Health Association, Chairman, Health and Medicine Policy Research Group, Chicago

October 8, 2009

UNRECOGNIZED CANCER AND HORMONAL RISKS OF AVON PRODUCTS

Chairman of the Cancer Prevention Coalition, Dr. Samuel Epstein, is warning women that toxic ingredients in Avon Products put users at risk of cancer and hormonal changes.

For this reason, Dr. Epstein is urging the National Cancer Institute to terminate plans for a joint project with Avon until the company reformulates its products to replace all toxic ingredients with safe alternatives.

A class of ingredients in Avon products, parabens, has been shown to stimulate the growth of breast cancer cells in laboratory tests and parabens have been identified as possible causes of breast cancer, Dr. Epstein points out.

Used as preservatives, parabens mimic the hormone estrogen, which is known to play a role in the development of breast cancers.

Dr. Epstein is concerned about cancer-causing ingredients in all cosmetics and personal care products, but he is particularly concerned about Avon Products because of a newly announced collaboration with the National Cancer Institute, a US government agency.

In August 2009, the National Cancer Institute's (NCI) Cancer Biomedical Informatics Grid (caBIG) and the Love/Avon Army of Women announced that they intend to collaborate. Their objective is to develop a computerized initiative to recruit and study women in order to improve the prevention, diagnosis, and treatment of breast cancer.

Dr. Epstein acknowledges that this is an "important and worthy objective."

Dr. Susan Love is a well-known and leading national breast cancer surgeon. The Avon Foundation is a non-profit organization of Avon Products, a leading global beauty company. Avon is the world's largest direct seller and markets to women in over 100 countries through independent sales representatives.

Relating to a prominent advertisement by Avon Products in a November 2008 issue of the *New York Times*, Dr. Epstein identified a wide range of toxic ingredients in their products:

- Benzophenone-1 (hormonal and penetration enhancer) in Nail Experts Nail Brightener.
- Methylparaben (hormonal), ethylparaben (hormonal), and imidazolidinyl urea (cancer precursor) in Wash-Off Waterproof Mascara.
- Ceteareth-20 (cancer precursor), and disodium EDTA (penetration enhancer) in Advance Techniques Body Building Conditioner.
- PEG-80 sorbitan laurate, and PEG-10 rapeseed sterol (cancer precursors) in Anew Beauty Youth-Awakening Lipstick.

- "I communicated these disturbing concerns to Avon's chief scientific officer. However, she responded dismissively," Dr. Epstein said.

Dr. Epstein then informed Dr. Love of these concerns. She replied reassuringly, but non-responsively, to the effect that this information "could be used for future research by Love/Avon."

However, and of major concern, says Dr. Epstein, is persuasive evidence that has accumulated over the last decade, that parabens are readily absorbed through the skin, and that they pose powerful hormonal or estrogenic effects even at very low concentrations.

Parabens have shown to be readily absorbed through the skin of immature female rodents, and to stimulate premature uterine growth, Dr. Epstein observes.

Parabens have also been shown to stimulate the growth of breast cancer cells in laboratory tests, and incriminated as possible causes of breast cancer, he warns.

Dr. Epstein stresses that parabens are the commonest of all ingredients in cosmetics and personal care products. "As disturbingly, it has been estimated that women are exposed to high levels, as much as 50 milligrams of parabens daily, from cosmetics and personal care products," he points out.

An article in the September 10, 2009 issue of the Journal of Clinical Oncology, indicates that breast cancer patients may unknowingly be dosing themselves with estrogen by using topical moisturizers. The researchers report that the estrogenically active substances found in laboratory tests of 16 moisturizers were not mentioned in the product ingredient lists. The moisturizers tested were not identified by brand name.

Of additional and generally unrecognized concern is that other ingredients in Avon products, benzophenone, and EDTA, are "penetration enhancers." These facilitate their own absorption, and that of other toxic ingredients in any product, deeply through the skin.

Based on these considerations, Dr. Epstein is urging the National Cancer Institute to "insist that Avon reformulate its products to phase out all toxic ingredients and replace them by safe alternatives" before proceeding with the computerized initiative to recruit and study women to improve breast cancer prevention, diagnosis, and treatment.

If Avon is unwilling to do this, the NCI should terminate its relationship with the Love/Avon initiative, Dr. Epstein says.

The Cancer Prevention Coalition has written to Dr. John E. Niederhuber, the director of the National Cancer Institute, detailing and warning of the risk of cancer, and other risks of Avon cosmetics and personal care products.

Dr. Epstein says products containing these toxic ingredients could be subject to the Food and Drug Administration's Black Box warning as required by the 1938 Federal Food, Drug, and Cosmetic Act.

November 17, 2009

U.K. LEADS THE WAY IN BANNING TOXIC INGREDIENTS IN COSMETICS AND PERSONAL CARE PRODUCTS

The Cancer Prevention Coalition commends the UK's largest nationwide chain of health food shops, Holland & Barrett, for its recently announced ban on beauty products containing some toxic ingredients, but warns that products containing a wide range other toxic ingredients remain on the shelves.

On October 6th, Holland & Barrett announced that it would "ban hundreds of leading beauty products over claims they contain toxic ingredients" in their 525 stores nationwide.

Holland & Barrett announced that they have been working over the past year behind the scenes with suppliers to eliminate the use of these chemicals. As a result, they decided to reject certain well-known brands from their stores and reformulate all their own label products.

The main ingredients of concern to Holland & Barrett in this ban are a group of hormonal preservatives known as parabens, and an unrelated harsh detergent known as sodium lauryl sulfate.

Holland & Barrett has additional stores in the Republic of Ireland, in South Africa and in The Netherlands, where they use the trade name "De Tuinen."

Holland & Barrett is the first UK company to take this action, but it is not alone.

In mid-October, the giant retailer Morrisons, one of the nation's leading supermarket chains with over 400 stores, announced that it would shortly review concerns regarding the dangers of parabens.

Cancer Prevention Coalition Chairman Samuel S. Epstein, M.D. warns that numerous published scientific studies over the last two decades have shown that the parabens—methyl, ethyl, propyl, butyl, and benzyl—pose toxic estrogen-like effects.

"These vary widely, from the most potent, butyl, which is hormonal at levels 100,000 times lower than natural estrogen, to the less potent methyl," Dr. Epstein says.

"Parabens readily penetrate the skin of immature female rodents, from where they can pass directly into the blood, and stimulate premature uterine growth," he explains. "Even at very low concentrations, parabens have also been shown to stimulate the growth of estrogen-sensitive breast cancer cells in laboratory tests," Dr. Epstein emphasizes. "Of additional concern, administering parabens to immature male rats decreases their sperm counts and testosterone levels.... Parabens have been identified in the breast tissue of a woman with breast cancer, presumably originating from its presence in a product used as an underarm deodorant or antiperspirant," he cautions, saying, "This incriminates parabens as a possible cause of breast cancer."

Sodium lauryl sulfate is a well-known harsh detergent and a penetration enhancer. Dr. Epstein explains that this chemical damages the superficial layers of the skin and causes prolonged damage to the skin barrier. This allows the ready penetration of carcinogens and other toxic ingredients in cosmetics and personal care products through the skin.

Evidence on the danger of parabens and sodium lauryl sulfate is still denied in the Cosmetic Ingredients Review's annual US Compendium. This document details the industry's claims on the safety of about 1,470 ingredients listed on the labels of cosmetic and personal care products, including parabens and sodium lauryl sulfate.

These two ingredients continue to be claimed "safe" in the *2009 Cosmetic Ingredients Review Compendium*, an annual publication of The Personal Care Products Council, formerly The Cosmetic Toiletry and Fragrance Association.

The Council also assures that all products that US consumers buy are safe, and under control. This reassurance remains in the Council's 2009 annual Cosmetic Ingredient Review Compendium.

Dr. Epstein cautions that the Council maintains dozens of full-time lobbyists at the federal and state levels, and pursues an aggressive political agenda against what it considers to be "unreasonable or unnecessary labeling or warning requirements."

"Holland & Barrett is to be commended for its initiative in phasing out parabens and sodium lauryl sulfate," says Dr. Epstein. "However, the company appears strangely unaware of other toxic ingredients. These include a wide range of other hormonal ingredients, such as phthalates and bisphenol, besides a still wider range of carcinogens."

November 24, 2009

RISKS OF MAMMOGRAPHY: HIDDEN ROLE OF THE AMERICAN CANCER SOCIETY

The series of recent articles on mammography which report the harm done by overscreening, written by *New York Times* columnist Gina Kolata, as well as in other newspapers, have made no reference to the hidden role of the American Cancer Society, warns Samuel S. Epstein, M.D., chairman of the Cancer Prevention Coalition.

Five radiologists have served as presidents of the American Cancer Society (ACS). In its every move, the ACS promotes the interests of the major manufacturers of mammogram machines and films, including Siemens, DuPont, General Electric, Eastman Kodak, and Piker.

This bias hypes mammography, which Dr. Epstein and Rosalie Bertell, Ph.D. of the International Physicians for Humanitarian Medicine emphasize is an avoidable cause of breast cancer.

"The mammography industry conducts research for the ACS and its grantees, serves on its advisory boards, and donates considerable funds," they warn. "DuPont also is a substantial backer of the ACS Breast Health Awareness Program; sponsors television shows and other media productions touting ACS literature for hospitals, clinics, medical organization, and doctors; produces educational films; and aggressively lobbies Congress for legislation promoting the nationwide availability of mammography services."

In virtually all its actions, the ACS has been and remains strongly linked with the mammography industry. Meanwhile, it ignores or attacks breast self examination (BSE), following training by expert nurses or clinicians, which is the safe and effective alternative, say Drs. Epstein and Bertell.

ACS promotion continues to lure women of all ages into mammography centers, leading them to believe that mammography is their best hope against breast cancer. A leading Massachusetts newspaper featured a photograph of two women in their twenties in an ACS advertisement that promised early detection results in a cure "nearly 100 percent of the time."

An ACS communications director, questioned by journalist Kate Dempsey, admitted in an article published by the Massachusetts Women's Community's journal Cancer, "The ad isn't based on a study. When you make an advertisement, you just say what you can to get women in the door. You exaggerate a point . . . Mammography today is a lucrative [and] highly competitive business."

Not surprisingly, the prestigious Chronicle of Philanthropy, the leading charity watch dog, has warned that the ACS "is more interested in accumulating wealth than saving lives."

This evidence on the complicity of the ACS was made available to Gina Kolata at her request on October 20th, Dr. Epstein says. However, in her subsequent series of articles, she made no reference to the role of the ACS in concealing the dangers of mammography from the nation's women.

Routine mammography delivers an unrecognized high dose of radiation, warn Drs. Epstein and Bertell. If a woman follows the current guidelines for premenopausal screening, over a 10 year period she would receive a total dosage of about 5 rads. This approximates the level of exposure to radiation of a Japanese woman one mile from the epicenter of atom bombs dropped on Hiroshima or Nagasaki.

"Mammography is a striking paradigm of the capture of unsuspecting women by run-away powerful technological and global pharmaceutical industries, with the complicity of the cancer establishment, particularly the ACS, and the rollover mainstream media," they warn.

Drs. Epstein and Bertell emphasize, "Promotion of the multibillion dollar mammography screening industry has also become a diversionary flag around which legislators and women's product corporations can rally, protesting how much they care about women, while studiously avoiding any reference to avoidable risks of breast cancer.

Screening mammography should be phased out in favor of annual clinical breast examination, (CBE), by a trained nurse and monthly breast self examination (BSE), also following training by a trained nurse. This is an effective, safe, and low-cost alternative, to diagnostic mammography, the two experts advise.

"Such action is all the more critical and overdue in view of the still poorly recognized evidence that mammography does not lead to decreased breast cancer mortality," they say.

Drs. Epstein and Bertell envision nationwide networks of BSE and CBE clinics, staffed by trained nurses, saying, "These low-cost clinics would also empower women by providing them with scientific evidence on the risks of breast cancer, and also on its prevention."

This information is of particular importance, they say, in view of the high incidence of breast cancer, which has increased by 18% from 1975, in spite of the multi-billion dollar US insurance and Medicare costs of mammography. Such funds should be diverted to establishing BSE clinics nationwide and providing public information on the wide range of avoidable causes of breast cancer.

This information was detailed in 2001 in a scientific article on "The Dangers and Unreliability of Mammography: Breast Examination As A Safe Effective and Practical Alternative," published in the prestigious *International Journal of Health Services* as long ago as 2001. This was co-authored by Dr. Epstein, Dr. Bertell, a leading international expert on radiation hazards, and the late Barbara Seaman, the leader and founder of the women's breast cancer movement.

ENDORSER:
Rosalie Bertell, PhD, Former President of the International Institute of Concern for Public Health, Toronto, Canada, Regent of the International Physicians for Humanitarian Medicine, Geneva, Switzerland

December 16, 2009

RECKLESS INDIFFERENCE OF THE AMERICAN CANCER SOCIETY TO CANCER PREVENTION

Early this month, top Republican Senator Charles E. Grassley sent letters to the American Cancer Society (ACS), besides the American Medical Association (AMA) and 31 other medical advocacy groups, asking them to provide detailed information on tax-deductible funds that they have received from drug and device makers. Such funds have encouraged these organizations to lobby on behalf of a wide range of industries and strongly influence public policy.

Senator Grassley also invited involvement of "whistleblowers interested in establishing communication regarding wrongdoing or misuse of public dollars." However, this wrongdoing still remains unrecognized by policy makers, let alone by the public. As a result, the incidence of a wide range of avoidable cancers has continued to escalate. Meanwhile, well-documented scientific information on their well-documented causes remains undisclosed or ignored by the ACS. (Epstein, S.S. Cancer Gate: How To Win The Losing Cancer War, 2005):

1971 The ACS refused to testify at Congressional hearings requiring FDA to ban the intramuscular injection of diethylstilbestrol, a synthetic estrogenic hormone, to fatten cattle, despite unequivocal evidence of its carcinogenicity, and the cancer risks of eating hormonal meat. Not surprisingly, US meat is banned by other nations worldwide.

1977 The ACS opposed regulating black or dark brown hair dyes, based on paraphenylenediamine in spite of clear evidence of its risks of non-Hodgkins lymphoma, besides other cancers.

1978 Tony Mazzocchi, then senior international union labor representative, protested that "Occupational safety standards have received no support from the ACS." This has resulted in the increasing incidence of a wide range of avoidable cancers.

1978 Cong. Paul Rogers censured ACS for its failure to support the Clean Air Act in order to protect interests of the automobile industry

1982 The ACS adopted restrictive cancer policies, rejecting evidence based on standard rodent tests, which are widely accepted by governmental agencies worldwide and also by the International Agency for Research on Cancer.

1984 The ACS created the industry-funded October National Breast Cancer Awareness Month to falsely assure women that "early (mammography) detection results in a cure nearly 100 percent of the time." Responding to question, ACS admitted: "Mammography today is a lucrative [and] highly competitive business." Also, the Awareness Month ignores substantial information on avoidable causes of breast cancer.

1992 The ACS supported the Chlorine Institute in defending the continued use of carcinogenic chlorinated pesticides, despite their environmental persistence and carcinogenicity.

1993 Anticipating the Public Broadcast Service (PBS) *Frontline* special "In Our Children's Food," the ACS trivialized pesticides as a cause of childhood cancer and charged PBS with "junk science." The ACS went further by questioning, "Can we afford the PBS?"

1994 The ACS published a highly flawed study designed to trivialize cancer risks from the use of dark hair dyes.

1998 The ACS allocated $330,000, under 1 percent of its then $680 million budget, to claimed research on environmental cancer.

1999 The ACS trivialized risks of breast, colon and prostate cancers from consumption of rBGH genetically modified milk. Not surprisingly, US milk is banned by other nations worldwide.

2002 The ACS announced its active participation in the "Look Good ... Feel Better Program," launched in 1989 by the Cosmetic Toiletry and

Fragrance Association, to "help women cancer patients restore their appearance and self-image during chemotherapy and radiation treatment." This program was partnered by a wide range of leading cosmetics industries, which failed to disclose information on the carcinogenic, and other toxic ingredients in their products donated to unsuspecting women.

2002 The ACS reassured the nation that carcinogenicity exposures from dietary pesticides, "toxic waste in dump sites, "ionizing radiation from "closely controlled" nuclear power plants, and non-ionizing radiation, are all "at such low levels that cancer risks are negligible." ACS indifference to cancer prevention became embedded in national cancer policy, following the appointment of Dr. Andrew von Eschenbach, ACS Past President-Elect, as director of the National Cancer Institute (NCI).

2005 The ACS indifference to cancer prevention other than smoking, remains unchanged, despite the escalating incidence of cancer, and its $1 billion budget.

Some of the more startling realities in the failure to prevent cancers are illustrated by their soaring increases from 1975 to 2005, when the latest NCI epidemiological data are available. These include:

- Malignant melanoma of the skin in adults has increased by 168 percent due to the use of sunscreens in childhood that fail to block long wave ultraviolet light;
- Thyroid cancer has increased by 124 percent due in large part to ionizing radiation;
- Non-Hodgkin's lymphoma has increased 76 percent due mostly to phenoxy herbicides; and phenylenediamine hair dyes;
- Testicular cancer has increased by 49 percent due to pesticides; hormonal ingredients in cosmetics and personal care products; and estrogen residues in meat;
- Childhood leukemia has increased by 55 percent due to ionizing radiation; domestic pesticides; nitrite preservatives in meats, particularly hot dogs; and parental exposures to occupational carcinogens;
- Ovary cancer (mortality) for women over the age of 65 has increased by

47 percent in African American women and 13 percent in Caucasian women due to genital use of talc powder;

- Breast cancer has increased 17 percent due to a wide range of factors. These include: birth control pills; estrogen replacement therapy; toxic hormonal ingredients in cosmetics and personal care products; diagnostic radiation; and routine premenopausal mammography, with a cumulative breast dose exposure of up to about five rads over ten years.

MAJOR CONFLICTS OF INTEREST

Public Relations

- 1998–2000: PR for the ACS was handled by Shandwick International, whose major clients included R. J. Reynolds Tobacco Holdings.
- 2000–2002: PR for the ACS was handled by Edelman Public Relations, whose major clients included Brown & Williamson Tobacco Company, and the Altria Group, the parent company of Philip Morris, Kraft, and fast food and soft drink beverage companies. All these companies were promptly dismissed once this information was revealed by the Cancer Prevention Coalition.

Industry Funding

ACS has received contributions in excess of $100,000 from a wide range of "Excalibur Donors," many of whom continue to manufacture carcinogenic products. These include:

- Petrochemical companies (DuPont; BP; and Pennzoil)
- Industrial waste companies (BFI Waste Systems)
- Junk food companies (Wendy's International; McDonalds's; Unilever/ Best Foods; and Coca-Cola)
- Big Pharma (AstraZenceca; Bristol Myers Squibb; GlaxoSmithKline; Merck & Company; and Novartis)
- Biotech companies (Amgen; and Genentech)
- Cosmetic companies (Christian Dior; Avon; Revlon; Elizabeth Arden; and Estee Lauder)
- Auto companies (Nissan; General Motors)

Nevertheless, as reported in the December 8, 2009 *New York Times*, the ACS responded that it "holds itself to the highest standards of transparency and public accountability, and we look forward to working with Senator Grassley to provide the information he requested."

THE CHRONICLE OF PHILANTHROPY

As the nation's leading charity watch dog, the Chronicle has warned against the transfer of money from the public purse to private hands. It also warned that "The ACS is more interested in accumulating wealth than in saving lives."

A copy of this release has been sent to Senator Charles E. Grassley, of Iowa.

January 15, 2010

AN FDA BAN ON GENETICALLY-ENGINEERED MILK IS TWENTY YEARS OVERDUE

In May 2007, Samuel S. Epstein, MD, Chairman of the Cancer Prevention Coalition, and other leading national experts on genetically-engineered, bovine growth hormone (rBGH) milk filed a Petition to the Food and Drug Administration (FDA), " Seeking the Withdrawal of the New Animal Drug Application Approval for Posilac®-Recombinant Bovine Growth Hormone (rBGH)."

In the absence of any response, on January 12, 2010, Dr. Epstein resubmitted this Petition to Michael Taylor, Deputy Commissioner of the Food and Drug Administration, again without any response.

This Petition requests the Secretary of Health and Human Services, and the Commissioner of Food and Drugs to suspend the approval of rBGH, a genetically engineered bovine growth hormone, and require milk and other dairy products produced with its use to be labeled with a warning such as, "Produced with the use of rBGH, and contains elevated levels of insulin-like growth factor, IGF-1, which poses major risks of breast, prostate, and colon cancers."

STATEMENT OF GROUNDS

The Veterinary Toxicity Of rBGH

Evidence of these toxic effects was first detailed in confidential Monsanto reports, based on records of secret nationwide rBGH veterinary trials, submitted to the FDA prior to October 1989 when they were leaked to one of the petitioners, Dr. Epstein. He then made these reports available to Congressman John Conyers, Chairman of the House Committee on Government Operations. On May 8, 1990, Congressman Conyers issued the following statement, "I find it reprehensible that Monsanto and the FDA have chosen to suppress and manipulate animal health test data."

Details of these toxic effects were subsequently admitted by Monsanto, and by the FDA, and were disclosed on the drug's veterinary label (Posilac®) in November, 1993. These toxic effects include injection site lesions, a wide range of other toxic effects, and an increased incidence of mastitis requiring the use and antibiotics, with resulting contamination of milk.

Abnormalities In rBGH Milk

A January 1994 Monsanto Executive Summary on rBGH, claimed that "natural milk is indistinguishable" from rBGH milk, and that "there is no legal basis requiring its labeling." However, there are a wide range of well-documented abnormalities in rBGH milk. These include: reduction in short-chain fatty acid and increase in long-chain fatty acid levels; increase in levels of a thyroid hormone enzyme; contamination with unapproved drugs for treating mastitis; and frequency of pus cells due to mastitis.

Increased Levels Of Insulin-Like Growth Factor 1 (IGF-1) In rBGH Milk

A wide range of publications have documented excess levels of IGF-1 in rBGH milk, with increases ranging from four- to 20-fold. Based on six unpublished industry studies, FDA admitted that IGF-1 levels in rBGH milk were consistently and statistically increased, and that these were further increased by pasteurization. These increases were also admitted by the pharmaceutical company Eli Lilly, in application for marketing authorization in the European Community. It should also be noted that pasteurization of milk increases IGF-1 levels.

IGF-1 Is Readily Absorbed From The Intestine Into The Blood

IGF-1 is a small protein component known as a peptide. As such it is readily absorbed into the blood. It survives digestion, and has marked growth promoting effects following short-term feeding tests in rats.

Increased IGF-1 Levels In Milk Increase Risks Of Breast, Colon And Prostate Cancers

Increased levels of IGF-1 have been shown to increase risks of breast cancer in 19 scientific publications, risks of colon cancer in 10 publications, and prostate cancer in 7 publications.

Increased IGF-1 Levels Inhibit "Apoptosis"

Of critical importance is the fact that increased IGF-1 levels block natural defense mechanisms, known as apoptosis, against early submicroscopic cancers.

RBGH Increases Twinning Rates

An increased rate of twinning in cows injected with rBGH was admitted by Monsanto on its November 1993 Posilac® label, and the incidence of fraternal twins. Monsanto also admitted that it increases "and complications such as premature delivery, congenital defects and pregnancy-induced hypertension."

The International Ban On The Use And Imports Of US rBGH Dairy Products

Based on well-documented veterinary and public health concerns, in June 30, 1999, the United Nations Food Safety Agency, representing 101 nations worldwide, ruled unanimously not to endorse or set a safety standard for rBGH milk. Effectively, this has resulted in an international ban on US milk, approximately 20% of which is rBGH.

FDA Policy On Labeling rBGH Milk

The FDA continues to mislead dairy producers and consumers with regard to its requirement for labeling of rBGH milk, with its deliberately false claim that "No significant difference has been shown between milk derived from rBST-treated and non-rBST treated cows."

"In fact, rBGH milk continues to pose major cancer and other risks to the entire US population."

The 2007 Petition has been endorsed by four other leading experts on genetically-engineered, recombinant bovine growth hormone (rBGH) milk. We look forward to a response.

ENDORSERS:

Ronnie Cummins
National Director
Organic Consumers Association

John Kinsman
President
Family Farm Defenders

Arpad Pusztai, PhD, FRSE
Consultant Biologist
Scotland

Jeffrey Smith
Executive Director
Institute for Responsible Technology

February 25, 2010

FOOD AND DRUG ADMINISTRATION ADMITS MEDICAL RADIATION RISKS, BUT STILL IGNORES THE DANGERS OF MAMMOGRAPHY

On February 9, the Food and Drug Administration announced that it would take stringent action to regulate "the most potent forms of medical radiation," particularly those from increasingly popular CT scans. The FDA is to be commended for warning that such radiation is unsafe and equivalent to that about of 400 chest X-rays, 0.4 rads (radiation absorbed dose), and "can increase a person's lifetime cancer risk."

However, the FDA remains strangely unaware that radiation from routine premenopausal mammography poses significant and cumulative risks of breast cancer. This is also contrary to conventional assurances that radiation exposure from mammography is trivial, about 1/ 1,000 of a rad, and similar to just that from a chest X-ray. However, the routine practice of taking two films of each breast results in exposure of about 0.4 rads, focused on the breast rather than on the entire chest. Thus, premenopausal women undergoing annual screening over a ten-year period are exposed to a total of at least four rads for each breast, at least eight times greater radiation than FDA's "cancer risk" level. Such high radiation exposure approximates to that of Japanese women living approximately one mile away from the site of the Hiroshima atom bomb explosion.

This alarming information is not new. In 1972, the prestigious National Academy of Sciences warned that the overall risks of breast cancer increase by one percent for every single rad exposure. This totals a 10 percent risk from 10 years annual premenopausal mammography. This warning was emphasized in my 1978 *The Politics of Cancer*, "Whatever you may be told, refuse routine mammograms, especially if you are pre-menopausal. The x-rays may increase your chances of getting cancer."

A 1993 Swedish study involving 42,000 women showed that those under the age of 55 who received regular premenopausal mammography experienced a 29 percent greater risk of dying from breast cancer. Based on a detailed review of these and a wide range of other such studies, the late Dr. John Gofman, the leading international authority on medical radiation, published an analysis in his classic 1995 book, *Preventing Breast Cancer*. He stressed that medical radiation is probably the single most important cause of the modern breast cancer epidemic.

These warnings were further detailed in a 2001 article, with some 50 scientific references, "The Dangers and Unreliability of Mammography: Breast Self Examination As A Safe Effective and Practical Alternative," published in the prestigious *International Journal of Health Services*. This was co-authored by Dr. Rosalie Bertell, a leading international expert on the dangers of radiation, the late Barbara Seaman, founder and leader of the women's breast cancer movement, and myself. An analysis of several 1993 studies showed that women who regularly performed monthly breast self-examination (BSE), particularly following training by qualified nurses, detected their cancers much earlier than those who failed to do so. That most breast cancers are first recognized by women themselves was even admitted by the American Cancer Society (ACS) as early as 1985. "We must keep in mind that at least 90 percent of women who develop breast cancer discover the tumors themselves."

The *International Journal of Health Services* article further stressed that cancer risks from mammography are up to fourfold higher for the two percent of women who are silent carriers of a gene known as the A-T (ataxia-telangiectasia), and highly sensitive to the carcinogenic effects of radiation. This accounts for up to about 20 percent of all breast cancers diagnosed annually.

These wide range of concerns on the still unrecognized dangers of routine premenopausal mammography are critical, especially in view of the current high incidence of breast cancer. Disturbingly, this has increased by about twenty percent since 1975 in spite of routine premenopausal mammography, and its multi-billion dollar insurance costs. Such funds should instead be directed to establishing BSE training clinics nationwide.

Five radiologists have served as presidents of the ACS. In its every move, the ACS promotes the interests of the major manufacturers of mammography machines, particularly the latest digital machines. These are four times more expensive, but no more effective than the film machines.

The mammography industry conducts "research" for the ACS and its grantees, serves on its advisory boards, and donates considerable funds. In virtually all its actions, the ACS has been and remains strongly linked with the industry. An ACS communications director admitted the obvious in a 1999 article published by the Massachusetts Women's Community's journal Cancer. "Mammography today is a lucrative [and] highly competitive business."

Not surprisingly, the prestigious *Chronicle of Philanthropy*, the nation's leading charity watch dog, has warned the obvious. The ACS "is more interested in accumulating wealth than saving lives." A national boycott of the ACS is well overdue.

March 29, 2010

FRANK CONFLICTS OF INTEREST IN THE NATIONAL CANCER INSTITUTE

In March 2010, the White House nominated Nobel Laureate Harold Varmus as Director of the National Cancer Institute (NCI).

As a key advisor to President Obama's 2008 Presidential campaign, Varmus was subsequently appointed Co-Chairman of the President's Council of Advisors on Science and Technology. He was previously President of the New York Memorial Sloan-Kettering Cancer Center.

Varmus has a distinguished track record in basic research on cancer treatment. However, as emphasized by the Cancer Prevention Coalition, this is paralleled by lack of familiarity with mounting scientific evidence on cancer prevention. Two decades ago, he claimed, "You can't do experiments to see what causes cancer—it's not an accessible problem, and not the sort of thing scientists can afford to do—everything you do can't be risky."

In 1995, Varmus, then Director of the National Institutes of Health, struck the "reasonable pricing clause," protecting against exorbitant industry profiteering from the sale of drugs, developed with tax payer money. Varmus also gave senior NCI staff free license to consult with the cancer drug industry.

In this connection, the 2008 edition of Charity Rating Guide & Watchdog Report listed Dr. Varmus with a compensation package of about $2.7 million. This is the highest compensation of over 500 major non-profit organizations ever monitored.

As a past major recipient of NCI funds for basic genetic research, Varmus warned that "reasonable pricing" clauses, protecting against exorbitant industry profiteering from drugs developed with tax-payer dollars, were driving away private industry. So he struck these from agreements between industry and the NCI. As a consequence, Varmus eliminated any price controls on cancer drugs made at the tax-payer expense.

Illustratively, using taxpayers' money, NCI paid for the research and development of Taxol, an anticancer drug, later manufactured by Bristol-Myers Squibb. Following completion of clinical trials, an extremely expensive process in itself, the public paid again for developing the drug's manufacturing process. Once completed, NCI officials gave Bristol-Myers Squibb the exclusive right to sell Taxol at an inflationary price. As investigative journalist, Joel Bleifuss, warned in a 1995 *In These Times* article, "Bristol-Myers Squibb sells Taxol to the public for $4.87 per milligram, which is more than 20 times what it costs to produce." Taxol has been a blockbuster for Bristol-Myers, posting sales of over $3 billion since its approval in 1992, and accounting for about 40 percent of the company's sales.

Taxol was not the only drug involved in such funding practices. Bristol-Myers Squibb now sells nearly one-third of the approximately thirty-five cancer drugs currently available, often with highly inflated profits, and often developed with taxpayer funds. In 1995, Varmus, a past major recipient of NCI funds for basic genetic research, decided that "reasonable pricing" clauses, protecting against profiteering from drugs developed with taxpayer dollars, were driving away private industry. So he struck these from pricing clauses.

Taxol was not an isolated example. Taxpayers have funded NCI's research and development for over two-thirds of all cancer drugs now on the market. In a surprisingly frank admission, Samuel Broder, NCI Director from 1989 to 1995, stated the obvious: "The NCI has become what amounts to a government pharmaceutical company." Nobel Laureate Leland Hartwell, President of the Fred Hutchinson Cancer Research Center, endorsed Broder's criticism. He further stressed that most resources for cancer research are spent on "promoting ineffective drugs" for terminal disease. In this connection, Memorial Sloan-Kettering's Leonard Saltz estimated that the price for new biotech drugs "has increased 500-fold in the last decade." Furthermore, the US spends five times more than the U.K. on cancer chemotherapy per patient, although survival rates are similar.

As an expert in cancer treatment, Varmus appears unaware that almost 700 carcinogens, to some of which the public is periodically or regularly exposed, have been identified by independent scientists. He also seems to be unaware that the more cancer is prevented the less there is to treat.

On June 15, 2009, a letter to Congressional leaders urging drastic reform of the Obama Cancer Plan to mandate prevention, besides urging the annual publication of a public registry of carcinogens, was released by the five scientists listed below. This letter also listed seven cancers, summarized their avoidable causes, and their increasing incidence since 1975, based on 2005 NCI data:

- Malignant melanoma (mortality) of the skin in adults has increased by 168% due to the use of sunscreens in childhood that fail to block long wave ultraviolet light;
- Thyroid cancer has increased by 124% due in large part to ionizing radiation;
- Non-Hodgkin's lymphoma has increased by 76% due mostly to phenoxy herbicides; and phenylenediamine hair dyes;
- Testicular cancer has increased by 49% due to pesticides; hormonal ingredients in cosmetics and personal care products; and estrogen residues in meat;
- Childhood leukemia has increased by 55% due to ionizing radiation; domestic pesticides; nitrite preservatives in meats, particularly hot dogs; and parental exposures to occupational carcinogens;
- Ovary cancer (mortality) for women over the age of 65 has increased by 47% in African American women and 13% in Caucasian women due to genital use of talc powder;
- Breast cancer has increased by 17% due to a wide range of factors. These include: birth control pills; toxic hormonal ingredients in cosmetics and personal care products; diagnostic radiation; and routine premenopausal mammography, with a cumulative breast dose exposure of up to about five rads over ten years.

However, and as an expert in cancer treatment, Varmus was unlikely to be aware of such scientific evidence, which was not widely recognized until relatively recently.

Based on recent estimates by the National Institutes of Health, the total costs of cancer are about $219 billion each year. The annual costs to taxpayers of diagnosis and treatment amounts to $89 billion; the annual costs of premature death are conservatively estimated at $112 billion; and the annual costs due to loss of productivity are conservatively estimated at $18 billion. The human costs surely are of far greater magnitude. Much of these costs could be saved by cancer prevention.

These concerns regarding Dr. Varmus have been recognized and endorsed by the following leading national experts on cancer prevention:

Rosalie Bertell, Ph.D.
Regent, International Physicians for Humanitarian Medicine

Janette D. Sherman, MD
New York Academy of Science, 2009

Quentin D. Young, MD
Chairman, Health and Medicine Policy Research Group

May 4, 2010

CANCER PREVENTION COALITION URGED SUPPORT OF THE SAFE CHEMICALS ACT

The Cancer Prevention Coalition encouraged people to support the Safe Chemicals Act of 2010, introduced by Senator Frank Lautenberg (D-NJ) on April 15 this year. This amends the 1976 Toxic Substances Control Act by requiring manufacturers to prove the safety of chemicals before they are marketed. Of particular concern are carcinogens, to which the public remains dangerously exposed and uninformed.

In 1971, President Richard Nixon declared the national "war against cancer," and the National Cancer Act was passed. This charged the National Cancer Institute (NCI) "to disseminate cancer information to the public."

The 1971 Act also authorized the President to appoint the director of NCI and control its budget, thus bypassing the scientific and budgetary authority of the director of 26 other National Institutes of Health (NIH).

As a result of this anomaly, NCI's current $5.3 billion budget, 17% that of the entire NIH, remains beyond control of NIH's director.

This special status of the NCI was challenged in 2003 by the National Academy of Sciences, at hearings of the House Energy and Commerce, and also by the Senate Health, Education, Labor and Pensions Committees.

Furthermore, contrary to the specific requirements of the 1971 Act, the NCI has still failed to "disseminate cancer information to the public," and to warn the public of a wide range of avoidable causes of cancer.

The 1988 amendments to the National Cancer Program called for "an expanded and identified research program for the prevention of cancer caused by occupational or environmental exposure to carcinogens." However, these amendments have been and remain ignored by the NCI.

For over four decades, NCI policies have been and remain fixated on damage control—screening, diagnosis, treatment and related research. Meanwhile priorities for prevention, from avoidable exposures to carcinogens in air, water, consumer products, and the workplace have remained minimal.

To be sure, smoking remains the best-known and single largest cause of cancer, particularly lung cancer. However, while lung cancer incidence rates in men have declined by 20% over the past three decades, those in women have increased by 111%. But more importantly, non-smoking cancers—due to known chemical and physical carcinogens—have increased substantially since 1975.

Some of the more startling realities in the failure to prevent cancer are illustrated by their soaring increases. Examples include:

- Malignant melanoma of the skin in adults has increased by 168% due to the use of sunscreens in childhood that fail to block long wave ultraviolet light;
- Thyroid cancer has increased by 124% due in large part to ionizing radiation;
- Non-Hodgkin's lymphoma has increased 76% due mostly to phenoxy herbicides; and phenylenediamine hair dyes;
- Testicular cancer has increased by 49% due to pesticides; hormonal ingredients in cosmetics and personal care products; and estrogen residues in meat;
- Childhood leukemia has increased by 55% due to ionizing radiation; domestic pesticides; nitrite preservatives in meats, particularly hot dogs; and parental exposures to occupational carcinogens;

- Ovary cancer (mortality) for women over the age of 65 has increased by 47% in African American women and 13% in Caucasian women due to genital use of talc powder;
- Breast cancer has increased 17% due to a wide range of factors. These include: birth control pills; estrogen replacement therapy; toxic hormonal ingredients in cosmetics and personal care products; diagnostic radiation; and routine premenopausal mammography, with a cumulative breast dose exposure of up to about five rads over ten years. Reflecting these concerns, Representatives Debbie Wasserman-Schultz and Henry Waxman have introduced bills promoting educational campaigns, including teaching regular breast self examination to high school students.

Paradoxically the escalating incidence of cancer over the last thirty years parallels its sharply escalating annual budget, from $690 million in 1975 to $5.2 billion this year. Of this, a mere $314 million (6%) is claimed to be allocated to NCI's mission on "Cancer Prevention and Control."

However, in spite of well-documented evidence relating the escalating incidence of cancer to a wide range of avoidable carcinogenic exposures, the NCI remains "asleep at the wheel," and has recklessly refused to devote significant resources to prevention.

The NCI has also ignored proddings from Congress and independent scientific experts to develop a comprehensive registry of carcinogens. Worse still, the NCI has misled the public by claiming that most cancers are due to 'unhealthy behavior,' blaming the victim, despite overwhelming evidence to the contrary.

For instance, the NCI still claimed that 94% of all cancers are due to "unhealthy behavior," such as smoking, poor nutrition, inactivity, obesity and over exposure to sunlight, while a mere 6% are attributable to environmental and occupational exposures.

These estimates are based on those published in 1981 by the late U.K. epidemiologist Richard Doll. However, from 1976 to 1999, Doll had been a closet consultant to U.K. and US industries, including General Motors, Monsanto and the asbestos industry. Following revelation of these conflicts of interest, just prior to his death in 2002, Doll admitted that most cancers, other than those related to smoking and hormones, "are induced by exposure to chemicals often environmental."

Furthermore the NCI has touted the imminent success of new cancer treatments, but says these promises have seldom borne out, and have been widely questioned by the independent scientific community.

For instance, Nobel Laureate Leland Hartwell, President of the Fred Hutchinson Cancer Control Center, warned in 2004 that Congress and the public are paying NCI $4.7 billion a year, most of which is spent on "promoting ineffective drugs" for terminal disease.

Based on recent estimates by the National Institutes of Health, the total costs of cancer have now reached $228 billion a year. The annual costs to taxpayers of diagnosis and treatment amount to $93 billion; the annual costs of premature death are conservatively estimated at $116 billion; and the annual costs due to lost productivity are conservatively estimated at $19 billion. These are quantifiable and inflationary economic costs. The human costs surely are of far greater magnitude.

May 7, 2010
PROTECT CHILDREN'S HEALTH FROM TOXIC BPA

Chairman of the Cancer Prevention Coalition, Samuel S. Epstein, M.D. is urging public support for the recently introduced Toxic Chemicals Safety Act of 2010. This establishes a program to review and protect children from risks of toxic exposures, including Bisphenol-A (BPA), a cause of reproductive disorders in women, besides a common contaminant in consumer goods.

On March 30 this year, the Washington Post announced that the Environmental Protection Agency listed BPA as "a chemical of concern." The Post also noted that the US Food and Drug Administration (FDA) previously expressed "concerns about the chemical's hormonal effect on human health." However, the American Chemistry Council claims "that BPA is not a risk to the environment at current low levels."

BPA is widely used in polycarbonate bottles, such as baby products, besides adult personal care and cosmetic products, food can linings, microwave oven dishes, dental sealants, and also medical devices. There are also other recently recognized major sources of BPA. These include cash register and credit-card receipts, which are coated with microscopic powdered BPA, and which many of us handle daily.

A 2007 review of about 700 studies on BPA, published in the journal Reproductive Toxicology, found that the fetus and infants are highly vulnerable to the toxic hormonal effects of this ingredient, technically known as "endocrine disruptive."

Dr. Epstein cites an accompanying study by National Institutes of Health researchers in the same journal, reported uterine damage in newborn rodents exposed to levels of BPA comparable with those of normal human exposure. "This finding may also implicate BPA as a cause of reproductive tract disorders in women, after their earlier exposure as fetuses or infants," he warns.

Previous studies in the journal Endocrinology, and elsewhere, reported that BPA masculinizes the brain of female mice and feminizes the brain of male mice. Toxic effects of this hormone disrupter in pregnant women are evidenced in their infant baby boys by the reduction in the normal distance between their anus and genitals. This decrease in anogenital distance is also associated with a decrease in sperm production.

Based on such evidence, Health Canada declared BPA to be a "toxic chemical" in early 2008.

In addition to these toxic effects, exposure of pregnant rodents to BPA, at levels 2,000 times lower than the Environmental Protection Agency's "safe dose," resulted in sexual abnormalities in their offspring. Dr. Epstein warns that these abnormalities include an increased number of "terminal end buds" in breast tissue, which are associated with a subsequent high risk of breast cancer. However, an American Plastics Council spokesman claimed that the human relevance of these findings is only "hypothetical."

Dr. Epstein warns that BPA has also been found in human blood, placental and fetal tissue, and incriminated as a predisposing factor for prostate cancer. "The authors of this study also linked endocrine-dependent human cancers, such as breast cancer, to the minimal levels of BPA to which pregnant women are exposed," he says.

An August 2, 2007 consensus statement by several dozen scientists warned that BPA, even at very low exposure levels, is probably responsible for many human reproductive disorders.

A September 2008 publication, Endocrine-Related Cancer, by Dr. Gail Prins reviewed the substantial scientific evidence on the toxic hormonal effects of BPA, besides other endocrine disruptive chemicals (EDCs) in pregnant women. She concluded that children are highly sensitive to their toxic effects, particularly subsequent risks of prostate cancer.

In October 2008, Science Daily reported on an article on BPA called "A Plastic World," in a then pending special section on Environmental Research. Two other articles reported that fetal exposure to BPA disrupted the normal development of the brain and behavior in rats and mice. Other articles have also reported that BPA is massively contaminating the oceans and harming aquatic wildlife.

The June 2009 Endocrine Disruption Act authorized the National Institute of Environmental Health Science "to coordinate" research on hormone disruption to prevent exposure to chemicals "that can undermine the development of children before they are born and cause lifelong impairment of their health and function."

This bill was supported by public health, consumer and children's advocacy groups, and further strengthened by California's Senator Dianne Feinstein's legislation to ban BPA from food and beverage containers. Of major relevance, this legislation has also been endorsed by the April 2010 President's Cancer Panel On "Reducing Environmental Cancer Risk: What We Can Do Now," 2008–2009 Annual Report. This report further warns that "to a disturbing extent, babies are born pre-polluted."

There are safe alternatives to BPA. As emphasized in the Dr. Sam Epstein's 2009 book *Toxic Beauty*, the recent development of "green chemistry" has encouraged the phase-out of product packaging that relies on petrochemical plastic containers, particularly those containing BPA. These containers are now being replaced with biodegradable substitutes, including recycled paper. Such "green" packaging reduces energy use, greenhouse gases, and non-degradable or poorly degradable wastes currently disposed of in landfills.

In January this year, the FDA announced an "Update on BPA," with particular reference to its use in food packaging, plastic baby bottles, feeding cups, and metal containers, to avoid childhood exposure. However, FDA has still not taken any regulatory action to this effect. Meanwhile, Dr.

Epstein says, the industry's Cosmetic Ingredient Review Panel does not even make any reference to BPA in its annual "safety assessments."

On April 15, Congressmen Bobby Rush and Henry Waxman released a draft of the Toxic Chemicals Safety Act of 2010. The key provisions of this Act include establishment of a program to review and protect children from risks of toxic exposures, including BPA.

Dr. Epstein says, "The passage of this legislation is urgently needed in order to ban BPA from food packaging and other consumer products, especially to prevent any further childhood exposure."

ENDORSER:
Gail S. Prins, Ph.D.
Professor of Physiology and Urology
University of Illinois at Chicago College of Medicine

May 7, 2010

AMERICAN CANCER SOCIETY TRIVIALIZES CANCER RISKS: BLATANT CONFLICTS OF INTEREST

The May 6 report by the President's Cancer Panel is well-documented. It warns of scientific evidence on avoidable causes of cancer from exposure to carcinogens in air, water, consumer products, and the workplace. It also warns of hormonal risks from exposure to Bisphenol-A (BPA) and other toxic plastic contaminants, says Samuel S. Epstein, M.D., Chairman of the Cancer Prevention Coalition (CPC).

Concerns on avoidable causes of cancer have been summarized in a January 23, 2009 Cancer Prevention Coalition press release, endorsed by 20 leading scientists and public policy experts, who urged that President Obama's cancer plan should prioritize prevention. These concerns were further detailed in a June 15, 2009 press release. Warnings of the risks of BPA are also detailed in a May 6, 2010 CPC release.

Some of the more startling realities in the National Cancer Institute's (NCI) and the "non-profit" American Cancer Society's (ACS) long-standing failure to prevent a very wide range of cancers are illustrated by their soaring increases from 1975 to 2005.

These include:

- Malignant melanoma of the skin in adults has increased by 168 percent due to the use of sunscreens in childhood that fail to block long wave ultraviolet light;
- Thyroid cancer has increased by 124 percent due in large part to ionizing radiation;
- Non-Hodgkin's lymphoma has increased 76 percent due mostly to phenoxy herbicides; and phenylenediamine hair dyes;
- Testicular cancer has increased by 49 percent due to pesticides; hormonal ingredients in cosmetics and personal care products; and estrogen residues in meat;
- Childhood leukemia has increased by 55 percent due to ionizing radiation; domestic pesticides; nitrite preservatives in meats, particularly hot dogs; and parental exposures to occupational carcinogens;
- Ovary cancer (mortality) for women over the age of 65 has increased by 47 percent in African American women and 13 percent in Caucasian women due to genital use of talc powder;
- Breast cancer has increased 17 percent due to a wide range of factors. These include: birth control pills; estrogen replacement therapy; toxic hormonal ingredients in cosmetics and personal care products; diagnostic radiation; and routine premenopausal mammography, with a cumulative breast dose exposure of up to about five rads over ten years.

Criticisms by the American Cancer Society that the President's Cancer Panel's report exaggerates avoidable cancer risks, reflect reckless indifference, besides narrow self-interest, warns Dr. Epstein.

In 1993, the nation's leading charity watch dog, The Chronicle of Philanthropy, warned against the transfer of money from the public purse to the private hands of the American Cancer Society. The Chronicle also warned that, "The ACS is more interested in accumulating wealth than saving lives."

These warnings are fully supported by the track record of the ACS for well over the last four decades.

- 1971: The ACS refused to testify at Congressional hearings requiring

FDA to ban the intramuscular injection of diethylstilbestrol, a synthetic estrogenic hormone, to fatten cattle, prior to their entry into feedlots prior to slaughter, despite unequivocal evidence of its carcinogenicity, and the cancer risks of eating hormonal meat. Not surprisingly, US meat is outlawed by most nations worldwide.

- 1977: The ACS opposed regulating black or dark brown hair dyes, based on paraphenylenediamine, in spite of clear evidence of its risks of non-Hodgkins lymphoma, besides other cancers.

- 1978: Tony Mazzocchi, then senior international union labor representative, protested that "Occupational safety standards have received no support from the ACS." This has resulted in the increasing incidence of a wide range of avoidable cancers.

- 1978: Congressman Paul Rogers censured ACS for its failure to support the Clean Air Act in order to protect interests of the automobile industry.

- 1982: The ACS adopted restrictive cancer policies, rejecting evidence based on standard rodent tests, which are widely accepted by governmental agencies worldwide and also by the International Agency for Research on Cancer.

- 1984: The ACS created the industry-funded October National Breast Cancer Awareness Month to falsely assure women that "early (mammography) detection results in a cure nearly 100 percent of the time." Responding to question, ACS admitted: "Mammography today is a lucrative [and] highly competitive business." Also, the Awareness Month ignores substantial information on avoidable causes of breast cancer.

- 1992: The ACS supported the Chlorine Institute in defending the continued use of carcinogenic chlorinated pesticides, despite their environmental persistence and carcinogenicity.

- 1993: Anticipating the Public Broadcast Service (PBS) *Frontline* special "In Our Children's Food," the ACS trivialized pesticides as a cause of childhood cancer and charged PBS with "junk science." The ACS went further by questioning, "Can we afford the PBS?"

- 1994: The ACS published a highly flawed study designed to trivialize cancer risks from the use of dark hair dyes.

- 1998: The ACS allocated $330,000, under 1 percent of its then $680 million budget, to claimed research on environmental cancer.

- 1999: The ACS trivialized risks of breast, colon and prostate cancers from consumption of rBGH genetically modified milk. Not surprisingly, US milk is outlawed by most nations worldwide.

- 2002: The ACS announced its active participation in the "Look Good...Feel Better Program," launched in 1989 by the Cosmetic Toiletry and Fragrance Association, to "help women cancer patients restore their appearance and self-image following chemotherapy and radiation treatment." This program was partnered by a wide range of leading cosmetics industries, which recklessly, if not criminally, failed to disclose information on the carcinogenic, and other toxic ingredients in their products donated to unsuspecting women.

- 2002: The ACS reassured the nation that carcinogenicity exposures from dietary pesticides, "toxic waste in dump sites, "ionizing radiation from "closely controlled" nuclear power plants, and non-ionizing radiation, are all "at such low levels that cancer risks are negligible." ACS indifference to cancer prevention became further embedded in national cancer policy, following the appointment of Dr. Andrew von Eschenbach, ACS Past President-Elect, as NCI Director.

- 2005: The ACS indifference to cancer prevention other than smoking, remains unchanged, despite the escalating incidence of cancer, and its $ billion budget.

The ACS's indifference to cancer prevention also reflects major conflicts of interest with regard to public relations, Dr. Epstein emphasizes.

PUBLIC RELATIONS

- 1998–2000: PR for the ACS was handled by Shandwick International, whose major clients included R.J. Reynolds Tobacco Holdings.

- 2000–2002: PR for the ACS was handled by Edelman Public Relations, whose major clients included Brown & Williamson Tobacco Company, and the Altria Group, the parent company of Philip Morris, Kraft, and fast food and soft drink beverage companies. All these companies were promptly dismissed once this information was revealed by the CPC.

INDUSTRY FUNDING

The ACS's indifference to cancer prevention reflects major industry funding. ACS has received contributions in excess of $100,000 from a wide range of "Excalibur Donors," many of whom continue to manufacture carcinogenic products, points out Dr. Epstein.

These include:

- Petrochemical companies (DuPont; BP; and Pennzoil)
- Industrial waste companies (BFI Waste Systems)
- Junk food companies (Wendy's International; McDonalds's; Unilever/Best Foods; and Coca-Cola)
- Big Pharma (AstraZenceca; Bristol Myers Squibb; GlaxoSmithKline; Merck & Company; and Novartis)
- Biotech companies (Amgen; and Genentech)
- Cosmetic companies (Christian Dior; Avon; Revlon; Elizabeth Arden; and Estee Lauder)
- Auto companies (Nissan; General Motors)

Nevertheless, warns Dr. Epstein, in spite of this long-standing track record of flagrant conflicts of interest, as reported in the December 8, 2009 *New York Times*, the ACS responded that it "holds itself to the highest standards of transparency and public accountability."

May 25, 2010

PRESIDENT'S CANCER PANEL WARNS OF TOXIC EFFECTS OF BISPHENOL A

Bisphenol-A (BPA) is widely used as a plasticizer in polycarbonate baby bottles, besides adult personal care and cosmetic products, food can linings, microwave oven dishes, dental sealants and also medical devices. Other recently recognized major sources are cash register and credit-card receipts, which are coated with microscopic powdered BPA, and which many of us handle daily.

The 2010 President's Cancer Panel report explicitly cited BPA as a "chemical of concern," and warned that "more than 130 studies have linked

BPA to breast cancer, obesity, and other disorders." The Panel rejected the March 2009 Food and Drug Administration (FDA) safety assessment of BPA as "incomplete and unreliable because it failed to consider all the relevant scientific works." The Panel also warned that FDA's "safety assessment on BPA" had been rejected by a March 2009 consortium of independent experts from academia, government and industry. The Panel report further emphasized that "science at the FDA is deficient, and the Agency is not prepared to meet regulatory responsibilities."

The scientific evidence on the toxic effects of BPA is extensive. A 2007 review of about 700 studies on BPA, published in the journal *Reproductive Toxicology*, found that the fetus and infants are highly vulnerable to the toxic hormonal effects of this ingredient, technically known as "endocrine disruptive." An accompanying study by National Institutes of Health researchers reported uterine damage in newborn rodents exposed to levels of BPA, comparable with those of normal human exposure. This finding may also implicate BPA as a cause of reproductive tract disorders in women, after their earlier exposure as fetuses or infants.

Previous studies in the journal *Endocrinology*, besides elsewhere, reported that BPA masculinizes the brain of female mice and feminizes the brain of male mice. Toxic effects of this hormone disruptor in pregnant women are evidenced in their infant baby boys by the reduction in the normal distance between their anus and genitals. This decrease is also associated with a decrease in sperm production. Based on such evidence, Health Canada declared BPA to be a "toxic chemical" in early 2008.

In addition to these toxic effects, exposure of pregnant rodents to BPA, at levels 2,000 times lower than the Environmental Protection Agency's "safe dose," resulted in sexual abnormalities in their offspring. These include an increased number of "terminal end buds" in breast tissue, which are associated with a subsequent high risk of breast cancer. However, an American Plastics Council spokesman claimed that the human relevance of these finding is only "hypothetical."

BPA has also been found in human blood, placental and fetal tissue, and incriminated as a predisposing factor for prostate cancer. The authors of this study also linked endocrine-dependent human cancers, such as breast cancer, to the minimal levels of BPA to which pregnant women are exposed.

An August 2, 2007 consensus statement by several dozen scientists warned that BPA, even at very low exposure levels, is probably responsible for many human reproductive disorders.

A September 2008 publication, Endocrine-Related Cancer, by one of us (Dr. Gail Prins) reviewed the substantial scientific evidence on the toxic hormonal effects of BPA, besides other endocrine disruptive chemicals (EDC's) in pregnant women. She concluded that infants and children are highly sensitive to their toxic effects, particularly subsequent risks of prostate cancer.

In October 2008, Science Daily reported on an article on BPA called "A Plastic World," in a then pending special section on Environmental Research. Two other articles reported that fetal exposure to BPA disrupted the normal development of the brain and behavior in rats and mice. Other articles have also reported that BPA is massively contaminating the oceans and harming aquatic wildlife.

The June 2009 Endocrine Disruption Act authorized the National Institute of Environmental Health Science "to coordinate" research on hormone disruption to prevent exposure to chemicals "that can undermine the development of children before they are born and cause lifelong impairment of their health and function." This Bill was supported by public health, consumer and children's advocacy groups, and further strengthened by California's Senator Dianne Feinstein's legislation to ban BPA from food and beverage containers. Of major relevance, this legislation has also been endorsed by the April 2010 President's Cancer Panel On "Reducing Environmental Cancer Risk: What We Can Do Now," 2008–2009 Annual Report. This further warns that "to a disturbing extent, babies are born pre-polluted."

It should be emphasized there are safe alternatives to BPA. As emphasized in the author's 2009 Toxic Beauty book, the recent development of "green chemistry" has encouraged the phase-out of product packaging that relies on petrochemical plastic containers, particularly those containing BPA. These containers are now being replaced with biodegradable substitutes, including recycled paper. Such "green" packaging reduces energy use, greenhouse gases, and non-degradable or poorly degradable wastes currently disposed of in landfills.

In January this year, the FDA announced an "Update on BPA," with particular reference to its use in food packaging, plastic baby bottles, feeding cups, and metal containers, to avoid childhood exposure. Nevertheless, FDA has still failed to take any regulatory action to this effect. Meanwhile, the industry's Cosmetic Ingredient Review Panel does not even make any reference to BPA in its annual "safety assessments."

In March this year, Congressmen Bobby Rush and Henry Waxman released a draft of the Toxic Chemicals Safety Act of 2010. The key provisions of this Act include establishment of a program to review and protect children from risks of toxic exposures, including BPA. The passage of this legislation is urgently needed in order to ban BPA from baby bottles, food packaging and other consumer products, especially to prevent any further childhood exposure.

One month later, Senator Lautenberg introduced the "Safe Chemicals Act of 2010," aimed at revamping the 34-year-old Toxic Substances Control Act. This is intended to ensure that "those who make the chemicals—ought to be responsible for testing them before they are released to the public." This surely should be the case for BPA.

June 16, 2010

RECKLESS FAILURE OF THE US FOOD AND DRUG ADMINISTRATION TO PROTECT AGAINST CANCER FROM TOXICS IN COSMETICS AND GE MILK

The Cancer Prevention Coalition reminds the American public that the 1938 Federal Food Drug and Cosmetic Act explicitly stipulates: "Each ingredient used in a cosmetic product and each finished cosmetic product shall be adequately substantiated for safety prior to marketing."

In the absence of adequate evidence of safety, products must be conspicuously labeled on their principle display panel: "WARNING: THE SAFETY OF THIS PRODUCT HAS NOT BEEN DETERMINED." Furthermore, the Food and Drug Administration (FDA) is authorized to pursue enforcement action after a product containing dangerous ingredients has been marketed.

However, warns Samuel S. Epstein, M.D., Chairman of the Cancer

Prevention Coalition, in spite of such explicit pre-and-post-marketing authority, the FDA has taken no regulatory action whatsoever over the last six decades, continuing until today, to protect the public from unknowing exposures to a wide range of toxic ingredients in cosmetic and personal care products. These include allergens, hormones, carcinogens and their precursors, and ultra-microscopic nanoparticles.

On November 17, 1994, the Cancer Prevention Coalition, the Ovarian Cancer Early Detection Prevention Foundation, and the Health and Medicine Policy Research Group filed a Citizens Petition to FDA Commissioner, David Kessler, M.D., on the dangers of talc, based on 17 scientific references dating back to the 1960's. These detailed evidence of major lethal risks of ovarian cancer, particularly in African-American women, from genital dusting with cosmetic grade talc. However, the Petition was rejected.

In May 2008, the Cancer Prevention Coalition, together with directors or representatives of six major national public health organizations, filed a further Petition to FDA Commissioner, Dr. Andrew von Eschenbach, based on additional more recent scientific evidence, "seeking a cancer warning on cosmetic talc products." However, the FDA was again unresponsive.

Not surprisingly, on September 10, 1997, Senator Kennedy warned that "the cosmetic industry has borrowed a page from the playbook of the tobacco industry." However, says Dr. Epstein, this is an understatement, as cigarette packs carry an explicit cancer warning, and smoking is uncommon until early adult life. In striking contrast, exposure to cosmetics and personal care products can be lifelong, following their use by pregnant women, and absorption of toxic ingredients through the skin, into the blood and then reaching the fetus.

On May 11, 2007, the Cancer Prevention Coalition, Organic Consumers Association, Family Farm Defenders, and Institute for Responsible Technology, filed a Citizens Petition to FDA Commissioner Andrew von Eschenbach, M.D., on the wide range of undisclosed dangers of genetically engineered bovine growth hormone, commonly known as rBGH, milk.

The Petition detailed the veterinary toxicity of rBGH. It also detailed the wide range of abnormalities in the composition of rBGH milk, particularly the 10-fold or more increased levels of a natural growth factor known as IGF-1, and its ready absorption from the small intestine into the blood; IGF-1 levels in milk are further increased by pasteurization.

"Drinking this milk results in major increased risks of colon, prostate, and breast cancers," Dr. Epstein emphasizes. "Increased IGF-1 levels also block natural defense mechanisms, known as apoptosis or programmed self-destruction, against early submicroscopic cancers. However, the FDA remains recklessly unresponsive to this Petition."

On January 12, 2010, the 2007 Citizen's Petition seeking the withdrawal of Posilac, the brand name under which rBGH is marketed, was re-filed to the current FDA Commissioner Margaret Hamburg, M.D. However, the FDA rejected this Petition, this time on the basis of alleged technical grounds, which had not been previously invoked.

"An even more recent example of FDA's irresponsibility," says Dr. Epstein, "has received prominent emphasis in the prestigious May 6, 2010 President's Cancer Panel (PCP) Report, with illustrative regard to bisphenol-A (BPA)." This ingredient is widely used as an unlabeled plasticizer in baby bottles and food containers, besides in cosmetics and personal care products.

The President's Cancer Panel explicitly warned that BPA "is a chemical of concern," and that "more than 30 studies have linked BPA to breast cancer, obesity, diabetes, and other disorders."

The President's Cancer Panel also summarily rejected, as "incomplete and unreliable," FDA's claims that bisphenol-A is safe, and the FDA's assertion "that neither a ban on the chemical or labeling of BPA-containing products was warranted."

Senator Frank Lautenberg's proposed "Safe Chemicals Act of 2010" would require manufacturers to provide information on "chemicals of concern" in consumer products. To say the least, this is timely, says Dr. Epstein. "Such information would provide the public with critical health and safety information on these products, especially as the FDA has failed to do so since passage of the 1938 Federal Food, Drug, and Cosmetic Act," he says. "Clearly, Congressional investigation and drastic reform of the FDA is decades overdue."

ENDORSERS:
Lennart Hardell, MD, PhD
Professor , Department of Oncology
University Hospital
Orebro, Sweden

Vicente Navarro, MD, PhD
Professor of Health Policy
The Johns Hopkins Medical Institutions

Janette D. Sherman, MD
Adjunct Professor Environmental Institute
Western Michigan University

Quentin D. Young, MD
Public Health Advocate, State of Illinois
Past President American Public Health Association
Chairman, Health and Medicine Policy Research Group

October 15, 2010

BREAST CANCER *UNAWARENESS* MONTH: RETHINKING MAMMOGRAMS

In 1984, the American Cancer Society (ACS), the world's largest nonprofit organization, inaugurated the October National Breast Cancer Awareness Month (NBCAM), with its flagship National Mammography Day. The NBCAM was conceived and funded by the Imperial Chemical Industries, a leading international manufacturer of petrochemicals, and its US subsidiary Zeneca Pharmaceuticals. Zeneca is the sole manufacturer of tamoxifen, which has been widely used for treating breast cancer.

The NBCAM has assured women that "early (mammography) detection results in a cure nearly 100 percent of the time." More specifically, the NBCAM directed its claims for reducing the incidence and mortality of breast cancer through early detection by annual mammography starting at age 40. Moreover, mammograms can miss cancers in premenopausal women due to the density of their breasts, and also fail to detect cancers smaller than half an inch.

Still denied by the ACS is clear evidence that premenopausal mammography poses significant risks of breast cancer. The routine practice of taking two films annually for each breast results in approximately 0.5 rad (radiation absorbed dose) exposure. This is about 500 times the dose from a single chest X-ray and is broadly focused on the entire chest rather than narrowly on the breast. This is also 25 times higher than is allowed by the Environmental Protection Agency for whole-body radiation from local nuclear industries (0.02 rad). Moreover, the breast is the most sensitive organ to ionizing radiation.

As warned by the prestigious National Academy of Sciences in 1972 but still ignored by the ACS, the premenopausal breast is highly sensitive to the risks of cancer from mammography, as each rad exposure increases the risks of breast cancer by 1 percent. This results in a cumulative 10 percent increased risk for each breast following a decade of routine screening. This can also accounts for the 19-percent increased incidence of breast cancer since 1975. Not surprisingly, the prestigious US Preventive Task Force, supported by the National Breast Cancer Coalition, warned last year against routine premenopausal mammography. Also, not surprisingly, routine premenopausal mammography is practiced by no nation other than the US.

Risks of premenopausal mammography are some four-fold greater for the 2 percent of women who are carriers of the A-T gene (ataxia telangiectasia) and are highly sensitive to the carcinogenic effects of radiation. By some estimates, this accounts for up to 20 percent of all breast cancers diagnosed annually. Compounding these problems, missed cancers are common in premenopausal women due to the density of their breasts.

That most breast cancers are first recognized by women was admitted by the ACS in 1985. "We must keep in mind that at least 90 percent of the women who develop breast cancer discover the tumors themselves." Furthermore, an analysis of several 1993 studies showed that women who regularly performed breast self-examination (BSE) detected their cancers much earlier than women failing to examine themselves. The effectiveness of BSE, however, depends on training by skilled professionals, enhanced by an annual clinical breast examination. Nevertheless, in spite of such evidence, the ACS dismisses BSE, and claims that "no studies have clearly shown [its] benefit."

As reported in our 1999 publication in the *International Journal of Health Services*, an article in a leading Massachusetts newspaper featured a photograph of two women in their twenties. The article promised that early detection by mammography results in a cure "nearly 100 percent of the time." Questioned by journalist Kate Dempsey, an ACS communications director responded: "The ad isn't based on a study. When you make an advertisement, you just say what you can to get women in the door. You exaggerate a point—Mammography today is a lucrative [and] highly competitive business."

If all 20 million US premenopausal women submitted to annual mammograms, the minimal annual costs would be $2.5 billion. Such costs would be increased some fourfold if the industry, supported by radiologists, succeeds in its efforts to replace film machines, costing about $100,000, with high-tech digital machines, costing over $400,000, even in the absence of any evidence for their improved effectiveness.

With this background, it is hardly surprising that the National Breast Cancer Awareness Month neglects to inform women how they can reduce their risks of breast cancer. In fact, we know a great deal about its avoidable causes which remain ignored by the ACS. These include:

- Prolonged use of the Pill, and estrogen replacement therapy.
- Prolonged consumption of milk from cows injected with a genetically engineered growth hormone to increase milk production. This milk is contaminated with high levels of a natural growth factor, which increases risks of breast cancer by up to seven-fold.
- High consumption of meat, as it is contaminated with potent natural or synthetic estrogens. These are routinely implanted in cattle before entry into feedlots, about 100 days prior to slaughter, to increase muscle mass and profits for the meat industry.
- Prolonged exposure to a wide range of hormonal ingredients in conventional cosmetics and personal care products.
- Living near hazardous waste sites, petrochemical plants, power lines, and nuclear plants.

The enthusiastic and continuing support of premenopausal mammography by the ACS is hardly surprising in view of its major conflicts of interest that still remain unrecognized. Five radiologists have served as ACS presidents. In its every move, the ACS promotes the interests of the major manufacturers of mammogram machines and films, including Siemens, DuPont, General Electric, Eastman Kodak and Piker.

The mammography industry also conducts research for the ACS, serves on its advisory boards, and donates considerable funds. DuPont is also a substantial backer of the ACS Breast Health Awareness Program. It sponsors television shows touting mammography; produces advertising, promotional materials and literature for hospitals and doctor; and lobbies Congress for legislation promoting the availability of mammography. The ACS has been and remains strongly linked with the mammography industry, while ignoring or criticizing the value of breast self-examination, even following training by a qualified nurse or clinician.

The ACS conflicts of interest extend well beyond the mammography industry. The ACS has received contributions in excess of $100,000 from a wide range of "Excalibur (industry) Donors," who manufacture carcinogenic products. These include petrochemical companies (DuPont, BP and Pennzoil), Big Pharma (AstraZenceca, Bristol Myers Squibb, GlaxoSmithKline, Merck & Company and Novartis), and cosmetic companies (Christian Dior, Avon, Revlon and Elizabeth Arden).

ENDORSER:

Rosalie Bertell, PhD

Former President of the International Institute of Concern for Public Health, Toronto, Canada

Regent of the International Physicians for Humanitarian Medicine, Geneva, Switzerland

January 10, 2011
UNRECOGNIZED DANGERS OF FORMALDEHYDE

The Cancer Prevention Coalition today is drawing public attention to a two page article in the *New York Times*, "When Wrinkle-Free Clothing Also Means Formaldehyde Fumes," published on December 10, 2010, which stated that "formaldehyde is commonly found in a broad range of consumer products." These include sheets, pillow cases, and drapes, besides "personal care products like shampoos, lotions, and eye shadows."

Samuel S. Epstein, M.D., who chairs the Cancer Prevention Coalition, says, "The dermatologists and other scientists quoted in the *Times* appear unaware of the longstanding scientific evidence on the carcinogenicity of formaldehyde. However, this had been detailed in five National Toxicology Program Reports on Carcinogens from 1981 to 2004."

The Times assured its readers that "most of the 180 items tested, largely clothes and bed linens, had low or undetectable levels of formaldehyde that met voluntary industry guidelines." Accordingly, the *Times* claimed, "Most consumers will probably never have a problem with exposure to formaldehyde," since such low levels "are not likely to irritate most people," other than those wearing wrinkle-resistant clothing.

However, Dr. Epstein points to evidence that links formaldehyde exposure with increased incidence of nasal cancer and breast cancer.

The Times article stated that "The US does not regulate formaldehyde levels in clothing. . . . Nor does any government agency require manufacturers to disclose the use of this chemical on labels."

But that could change. On March 5, 2008, Senators Bob Casey, Sherrod Brown, and Mary Landrieu introduced an amendment to the Consumer Product Safety Commission (CPSC) reform bill "that would help protect Americans from dangerous levels of formaldehyde in textiles including clothing . . ."

The Senators referred to a 1997 CPSC report on formaldehyde, which admitted that "it causes cancer in tests on laboratory animals, and may cause cancer in humans." Accordingly, the Senators requested the CPSC to "regulate and test formaldehyde in textiles—and protect consumers from this poison."

In August 2010, a Government Accountability Office (GAO) report warned that "a small proportion of the US population does have allergic reactions to formaldehyde resins on their clothes." However, the GAO made no recommendations for any regulatory action.

Dr. Epstein supports both regulatory and legislative action based on scientific evidence in the five National Toxicology Program Reports on Carcinogens that classified formaldehyde as "reasonably anticipated to be a human carcinogen," based on limited evidence of carcinogenicity in humans, and sufficient evidence in experimental animals.

This evidence was confirmed in a series of reports by the prestigious

International Agency for Research on Cancer (IARC). Its 2006 and 2010 reports explicitly warn that formaldehyde is "a known cause of leukemia in experimental animals—and nasal cancer" in humans.

"Strong" evidence of the nasal cancer risk was also cited in the May 2010 President's Cancer Panel report, "Environmental Cancer Risk: What Can We Do Now?"

"Nevertheless," says Dr. Epstein, "and in spite of this explicit evidence, a September 2010 Government Accountability Office report attempted to trivialize the cancer risks of formaldehyde on the alleged grounds that exposure levels are low or 'non-detectable.'"

Of further concern, Dr. Epstein warns, "occupational exposure to formaldehyde has been associated with breast cancer deaths in a 1995 National Cancer Institute report, while environmental exposure has been associated with an increased incidence of breast cancer in a 2005 University of Texas report."

"Disturbingly," observes Dr. Epstein, "none of the dermatologists quoted in the *New York Times* appear aware of longstanding evidence that most cosmetics and personal care products, commonly used daily by most women, besides on their infants and children, and to a lesser extent men, contain up to eight ingredients which are precursors of formaldehyde."

These include diazolidinyl urea, metheneamine, and quaterniums, each of which readily breaks down on the skin to release formaldehyde, Dr. Epstein explains, warning, "This is then readily absorbed through the skin, and poses unknowing risks of cancer to most of the US population."

March 14, 2011
THE AMERICAN CANCER SOCIETY: "MORE INTERESTED IN ACCUMULATING WEALTH THAN SAVING LIVES"

My March 14, 2011 report on the American Cancer Society (ACS), "More Interested In Accumulating Wealth Than Saving Lives" was released. This report was endorsed by Congressman John Conyers Jr., Chairman of the House Judiciary Committee, and Quentin Young M.D., Chairman of the Health and Medicine Policy research Group, and Past President of the

American Public Health Association.

The report traces the track record of the ACS, since its founding in 1913 by a group of oncologists and wealthy business men until this year. It documents the virtually exclusive priority of the ACS to the diagnosis and treatment of cancer, with indifference to prevention, other than that due to faulty personal lifestyle. Commonly known as "blame the victim," this excludes the very wide range of scientifically well-documented avoidable causes of cancer.

The ACS track record clearly reflects frank conflicts of interest. About half the ACS board are clinicians, oncologists, surgeons, and radiologists, mostly with close ties to the National Cancer Institute (NCI). Many board members and their institutional colleagues apply to and obtain funding from both the ACS and the NCI. Substantial NCI funds also go to ACS directors who sit on key NCI committees. Although the ACS asks its board members to leave the room when others review their funding proposals, this is just a token formality. In this private club, easy access to funding is one of the perks, as the board routinely rubber-stamps approvals. A significant amount of ACS funding also goes to this extended membership. Frank conflicts of interest are also evident in many ACS priorities. These include policies on mammography, the National Breast Cancer Awareness campaign, and the pesticide and cancer drug industries. These conflicts extend to the virtual privatization of national cancer policy.

For instance the ACS has close connections to the mammography industry. Five radiologists have served as ACS presidents. In its every move, the ACS reflects the interests of the major manufacturers of mammography, films and machines. These include Siemens, DuPont, General Electric, Eastman Kodak, and Piker, which allocate considerable funds to the ACS.

ACS promotion still continues to lure women of all ages into mammography centers, leading them to believe that mammography is their best hope against breast cancer. An ACS advertisement in a leading Massachusetts newspaper featured a photograph of two women in their twenties that recklessly promised that early detection results in a cure "nearly 100 percent of the time." An ACS communications director, questioned by journalist Kate Dempsey, responded in an article published by the Massachusetts Women's Community's journal *Cancer*: "The ad isn't based on a study. When you make an advertisement, you just say what you can to get women in the door. You exaggerate a point. Mammography today is a lucrative [and] highly competitive business." However, the National Academy of Science has warned that the premenopausal breast is highly sensitive to radiation, and that annual mammography can increase risks of breast cancer by 10%. Furthermore, the US Preventive Task Force, supported by the National Breast Cancer Coalition, has recently recommended that routine mammography should be delayed until the age of 50 and practiced every 2 years subsequently until the age of 75.

The ACS has also had a strong relation with a wide range of industries, including the pesticide and cancer drug. Responding to concerns on risks on carcinogenic pesticides in food, the ACS responded, "We have no cancer cases in which pesticide use was confirmed as the cause." Also referring to concerns on the multibillion dollar cancer drug industry sales, the ACS dismisses "unproven," non-patentable and minimally toxic alternatives. This claim however is in the striking contrast to its hidden conflicts of interest.

Public Relations

1998-2000: PR for the ACS was handled by Shandwick International, whose major clients included R.J. Reynolds Tobacco Holdings.

2000-2002: PR for the ACS was handled by Edelman Public Relations, whose major clients included Brown & Williamson Tobacco Company, and Altria Group, the parent company of Philip Morris, Kraft, and fast food and soft drink beverage companies. All these companies were preemptively dismissed once this information was revealed by the Cancer Prevention Coalition.

Industry Funding

ACS has received contributions in excess of $100,000 from a wide range of "Excalibur Donors." Some of these companies were responsible for environmental pollution with carcinogens, while others manufactured and sold products containing toxic and carcinogenic ingredients. These include:

- Petrochemical companies (DuPont; BP; and Pennzoil)
- Industrial waste companies (BFI Waste Systems)
- Big Pharma (AstraZeneca; Bristol Myers Squibb; GlaxoSmithKline; Merck & Company; and Novartis)

- Auto companies (Nissan; and General Motors)
- Cosmetic companies (Christian Dior; Avon; Revlon; and Elizabeth Arden)
- Junk food companies (Wendy's International; McDonalds's; Unilever/ Best Foods; and Coca-Cola)
- Biotech companies (Amgen; and Genentech)

Nevertheless, as reported in the December 8, 2009 *New York Times*, the ACS claimed that it "holds itself to the highest standards of transparency and public accountability." Of major concern is the reckless record of the ACS with regard to cancer prevention over the past four decades.

1971 When studies unequivocally proved that diethylstilbestrol (DES) caused vaginal cancers in teenage daughters of women administered the drug during pregnancy, the ACS refused an invitation to testify at Congressional hearings to require the Food and Drug Administration to ban its use as an animal feed additive. It gave no reason for its refusal. Not surprisingly, US meat is banned by other nations worldwide.

1983 The ACS refused to join a coalition of the March of Dimes, American Heart Association, and the American Lung Association in support of the Clean Air Act.

1992 The ACS issued a joint statement with the Chlorine Institute in support of the continued global use of organochlorine pesticides, despite clear evidence that some of these were known to cause breast cancer. In this statement, ACS vice president Clark Heath, M.D., dismissed the evidence of any risk as "preliminary and mostly based on a weak and indirect association."

1993 Just before PBS *Frontline* aired the special entitled, "In Our Children's Food," the ACS came out in support of the pesticide industry. In a damage-control memorandum sent to some 48 regional divisions and their 3,000 local offices, the ACS trivialized pesticides as a cause of childhood cancer. The ACS also reassured the public that carcinogenic pesticide residues in food are safe, even for babies.

1994 The ACS published a study designed to reassure women on the safety of dark permanent hair dyes, and to trivialize risk of fatal and non-fatal cancers, particularly non-Hodgkin lymphoma, as documented in over six prior reports.

1999 The ACS denied any risks of cancer from drinking genetically-engineered (rBGH) milk. Its position has remained unchanged in spite of strong scientific decade old strong evidence relating rBGH milk to major risks of breast, prostate, and colon cancers.

2000 The Washington-Insider *Cancer Letter*, revealed that the ACS has close ties to the tobacco industry, notably Shandwick International, representing R.J Reynolds Tobacco Holdings, and subsequently Edelman Public Relations, representing Brown & Williamson Tobacco company.

2002 The ACS initiated the "Look Good...Feel Better" program to teach women cancer patients beauty techniques to help restore their appearance and self-image during chemotherapy and radiation treatment." This program was partnered by the National Cosmetology Association and The Cosmetic, Toiletry and Fragrance Association Foundation, which failed to disclose the wide range of carcinogenic ingredients in toiletries and cosmetics. These trade organizations also failed to disclose evidence of risks of breast and other cancers following long-term use of black or dark brown permanent and semi-permanent hair dyes. The ACS also failed to inform women of these avoidable risks. The Environmental Cancer Risk Section of the *ACS Facts and Figures Report* also reassured that carcinogenic exposures from dietary pesticides, "toxic wastes in dump sites"—are "all at such low levels that risks are negligible."

2007 The ACS indifference to cancer prevention, other than smoking, has remained unchanged despite its $1 billion budget, and despite the escalating incidence of cancer from 1975. This includes post menopausal breast cancer, 23%; childhood cancer, 30%; testis cancer 60%; and non-Hodgkin lymphoma, 82%.

2009 The ACS budget was about $1 billion, of which 17% was allotted to smoking cessation programs, and 28% to support services and salaries. The top three executive salaries ranged from $670,000 to $1.2 million.

2010 The ACS rejected the April 2010 President's Cancer Panel report, "Reducing Environmental Cancer." This had been widely endorsed by leading scientific and public policy experts. Nevertheless, the ACS brazenly claimed that more studies were needed to justify this conclusion.

The ACS track record of frank indifference to cancer prevention, other than that due to faulty lifestyle, extends to cancer organizations in Canada and 90 nations worldwide in support of their "Relay For Life" programs. Team members take turns to walk or run around a track for 12-24 hours. "Through the Relay, these organizations bring together passionate volunteers, to take action in the international movement to end cancer, by stopping smoking and developing healthy lifestyles. Funds raised by these Relays support local organizations' cancer control programs, services, and research." These organizations also contribute part of their funds to ACS "cancer control programs" worldwide.

Clearly the ACS continues to forfeit its public trust and support.

October 21, 2011

CORPORATE SPONSORS CONTROL MAMMOGRAPHY INDUSTRY

The Cancer Prevention Coalition says that National Mammography Day, the flagship event of National Breast Cancer Awareness Month (NBCAM), is a long overdue time to recognize the risks of mammography. Even more so, it is well past the time to recognize the links between the mammography and chemicals industries and the American Cancer Society.

National Breast Cancer Awareness Month was conceived and funded in 1984 by the American Cancer Society (ACS) and by the Imperial Chemical Industries (ICI) and its US subsidiary and spinoff Zeneca Pharmaceuticals.

Cancer Prevention Coalition chairman Samuel S. Epstein, M.D. says, "The NBCAM is a multi-million-dollar deal between the corporate sponsors and the National Cancer Institute (NCI) and the American Cancer Society."

"Mammography screening is a profit-driven technology posing risks compounded by unreliability," Dr. Epstein declares.

The American Cancer Society is knee deep in conflicts of interest with the mammography industry, says Dr. Epstein, who points out that five radiologists have served as ACS presidents. "In its every move, the ACS promotes the interests of the major manufacturers of mammogram machines and films, including Siemens, DuPont, General Electric, Eastman Kodak, and Piker," Dr. Epstein says.

The mammography industry also conducts research for the ACS, serves on its advisory boards, and donates considerable funds, says Dr. Epstein. DuPont also is a substantial backer of the ACS Breast Health Awareness Program, sponsors television shows and other media productions touting mammography, produces educational films, and lobbies Congress for legislation promoting availability of mammography services.

"In virtually all its important actions, the ACS has been and still remains strongly linked with the mammography industry, while ignoring or attacking the viable alternative of breast self examination (BSE)," says Dr. Epstein.

Imperial Chemical Industries is one of the largest manufacturers of petrochemical industrial chemicals, and Zeneca is the sole manufacturer of tamoxifen, the world's top selling cancer drug widely used for breast cancer.

"The ICI/Zeneca financial sponsorship gives them control over every leaflet, poster, publication, and commercial produced by NBCAM," warns Dr. Epstein.

"The ICI also supports the ACS blame-the-victim claim, which attributes escalating rates of breast along with other cancers to heredity and faulty lifestyle," he says. "This false and self-interested claim diverts attention away from avoidable exposures to carcinogenic industrial contaminants of air, water, food, consumer products, and the workplace."

DANGERS OF SCREENING MAMMOGRAPHY

"Radiation from routine premenopausal mammography poses significant cumulative risks of promoting breast cancer," Dr. Epstein warns.

"Contrary to conventional assurances that radiation exposure from mammography is trivial and similar to that of a chest x-ray, about 1/1000 of a rad (radiation absorbed dose), the routine practice of taking four films for each breast results in some 1,000-fold greater exposure, 1 rad, focused on each breast rather than on the entire chest," he explains. "Thus, premenopausal women undergoing annual screening over a 10-year period are exposed to a total of about 10 rads for each breast."

As emphasized some three decades ago, the premenopausal breast is highly sensitive to radiation, each rad exposure increasing breast cancer risk by 1 percent, resulting in a cumulative 10 percent increased risk over 10 years.

In striking contrast, annual clinical breast examination (CBE) by a trained health professional, in addition to monthly breast self-examination, is safe, at least as effective as mammography, and low, if any, in cost.

A national program for training nurses how to perform clinical breast examination, and also teach breast self examination, is critical and decades overdue, Dr. Epstein advises.

Mammography is not a technique for early diagnosis, contrary to popular belief and assurances by the ACS, and also the media. Dr. Epstein says that in fact, a breast cancer has usually been present for about eight years before it can be belatedly detected by mammography

THE MAMMOGRAPHY INDUSTRY

The ACS has close connections to the mammography industry, as Dr. Epstein detailed in his 1998 book, *The Politics of Cancer Revisited*. "In fact, if every woman followed ACS and NCI mammography guidelines, the annual revenue to health care facilities would be a staggering $5 billion," he says today.

"The ACS promotion continues to lure women of all ages into mammography centers, leading them to believe that mammography is their best hope against breast cancer," said Dr. Epstein.

He cites a leading Massachusetts newspaper that featured a photograph of two women in their twenties in an ACS advertisement that promised early detection results in a cure "nearly 100 percent of the time."

An ACS communications director, questioned by journalist Kate Dempsey, responded in an article published by the Massachusetts Women's Community's journal *Cancer*, saying, "The ad isn't based on a study. When you make an advertisement, you just say what you can to get women in the door. You exaggerate a point. Mammography today is a lucrative [and] highly competitive business."

Dr. Epstein warns that the ACS exposes premenopausal women to radiation hazards from mammography with little or no evidence of benefits. The ACS also fails to tell them that their breasts will change so much over time that the "baseline" images have little or no future relevance. This is truly an American Cancer Society crusade. But against whom, or rather, for whom?

THE AMERICAN CANCER SOCIETY'S CONFLICTS OF INTEREST

About half of the ACS board members are clinicians, oncologists, surgeons, radiologists, and basic molecular scientists, mostly with close ties to the NCI. Many board members and their colleagues apply for and obtain funding from both the ACS and the NCI. Substantial NCI funds also go to ACS directors who sit on key NCI committees. Although the ACS asks board members to leave the room when the rest of the board discusses their funding proposals, this is just a token formality. In this private club, easy access to funding is one of the perks as the board routinely rubber-stamps approvals. A significant amount of ACS research funding goes to this extended membership.

Frank conflicts of interest are evident in many ACS priorities. These include their advocating mammography and the National Breast Cancer Awareness campaign and supporting the pesticide and cancer drug industries. These conflicts even extend to the privatization of national cancer policy.

PUBLIC RELATIONS

- 1998–2000: PR for the ACS was handled by Shandwick International, whose major clients included RJ Reynolds Tobacco Holdings.

- 2000–2002: PR for the ACS was handled by the Edelman Public Relations, whose major clients included Brown & Williamson Tobacco Company, and the Altria Group, the parent company of Philip Morris, and Kraft.

INDUSTRY FUNDING

ACS has received contributions in excess of $100,000 from a wide range of "Excalibur donors." Some of these companies were responsible for environmental pollution with carcinogens while others manufactured and sold products containing toxic and carcinogenic ingredients.

These donors include:

- Petrochemical companies (DuPont, BP and Pennzoil)
- Industrial waste companies (BFI Waste Systems)
- Big Pharma (AstraZeneca, Bristol-Myers Squibb, GlaxoSmithKline, Merck & Company, and Novartis)
- Auto companies (Nissan and General Motors)
- Cosmetic companies (Christian Dior, Avon, Revlon, and Elizabeth Arden)
- Junk food companies (Wendy's International, McDonalds's, Unilever/ Best Foods, and Coca-Cola.
- Biotech companies (Amgen and Genetech)

October 28, 2011

THE NATIONAL MAMMOGRAPHY DAY

The National Mammography Day, October 21, is the flagship of the National Breast Cancer Awareness Month (NBCAM). This was conceived and funded in 1984 by the American Cancer Society (ACS) and by the Imperial Chemical Industries (ICI) and its US subsidiary and spinoff Zeneca Pharmaceuticals. The NBCAM is a multimillion-dollar deal between the corporate sponsors and the National Cancer Institute (NCI) and ACS.

The ACS is knee deep in conflicts of interest with the mammography industry. Five radiologists have served as ACS presidents. In its every move, the ACS promotes the interests of the major manufacturers of mammogram machines and films, including Siemens, DuPont, General Electric, Eastman Kodak, and Piker. The mammography industry also conducts research for the ACS, serves on its advisory boards, and donates considerable funds. DuPont also is a substantial backer of the ACS Breast Health Awareness Program, sponsors television shows and other media productions touting mammography, produces educational films, and lobbies Congress for legislation promoting availability of mammography services. In virtually all its important actions, the ACS has been and still remains strongly linked with the mammography industry, while ignoring or attacking the viable alternative of breast self examination (BSE).

ICI is one of the largest manufacturers of petrochemical industrial chemicals, and Zeneca is the sole manufacturer of tamoxifen, the world's top selling cancer drug widely used for breast cancer. The ICI/Zeneca financial sponsorship gives them control over every leaflet, poster, publication, and commercial produced by NBCAM. The ICI also supports the ACS blame-the-victim claim, which attributes escalating rates of breast, besides cancers to heredity and faulty lifestyle. This false and self-interested claim diverts attention away from avoidable exposures to carcinogenic industrial contaminants of air, water, food, consumer products, and the workplace.

DANGERS OF SCREENING MAMMOGRAPHY

Radiation from routine premenopausal mammography poses significant cumulative risks of promoting breast cancer. Contrary to conventional assurances that radiation exposure from mammography is trivial and similar to that of a chest x-ray, about 1/1000 of a rad (radiation absorbed dose), the routine practice of taking four films for each breast results in some 1,000-fold greater exposure, 1 rad, focused on each breast rather than on the entire chest. Thus, premenopausal women undergoing annual screening over a ten-year period are exposed to a total of about 10 rads for each breast. As emphasized some three decades ago, the premenopausal breast is highly sensitive to radiation, each rad exposure increasing breast cancer risk by 1 percent, resulting in a cumulative 10 percent increased risk over ten years.

Mammography screening is a profit-driven technology posing risks compounded by unreliability. In striking contrast, annual clinical breast examination (CBE) by a trained health professional, besides monthly breast self-examination (BSE), is safe, at least as effective as mammography, and low, if any, in cost. A national program for training nurses how to perform CBE, and also teach BSE is critical and decades overdue.

However, and contrary to popular belief and assurances by the ACS, and also the media, mammography is not a technique for early diagnosis. In fact, a breast cancer has usually been present for about eight years before it can be belatedly detected.

THE MAMMOGRAPHY INDUSTRY

The ACS has close connections to the mammography industry. As detailed in my 1998 *The Politics of Cancer Revisited*, five radiologists have served as ACS presidents, and in its every move, the ACS reflects the interests of the major manufacturers of mammogram machines and films. These include Siemens, DuPont, General Electric, Eastman Kodak, and Piker. In fact, if every woman followed ACS and NCI mammography guidelines, the annual revenue to health care facilities would be a staggering $5 billion.

The ACS promotion continues to lure women of all ages into mammography centers, leading them to believe that mammography is their best hope against breast cancer. A leading Massachusetts newspaper featured a photograph of two women in their twenties in an ACS advertisement that promised early detection results in a cure "nearly 100 percent of the time." An ACS communications director, questioned by journalist Kate Dempsey responded in an article published by the Massachusetts Women's Community's journal *Cancer*: "The ad isn't based on a study. When you make an advertisement, you just say what you can to get women in the door. You exaggerate a point. Mammography today is a lucrative [and] highly competitive business."

In addition, the mammography industry conducts research for the ACS and its grantees, serves on advisory boards, and donates considerable funds. DuPont is a substantial backer of the ACS Breast Health Awareness Program; sponsors television shows and other media productions touting mammography; produces advertising, promotional, and educational literature and films for hospitals, clinics, medical organizations, and doctors; and lobbies Congress for legislation promoting availability of mammography services. In virtually all of these important actions the ACS remains strongly linked with the mammography industry while ignoring the development of viable alternatives to mammography, particularly breast self-examination.

The ACS exposes premenopausal women to radiation hazards from mammography with little or no evidence of benefits. The ACS also fails to tell them that their breasts will change so much over time that the "baseline" images have little or no future relevance. This is truly an American Cancer Society crusade. But against whom, or rather, for whom?

THE AMERICAN CANCER SOCIETY'S CONFLICTS OF INTEREST

About half of the ACS board members are clinicians, oncologists, surgeons, radiologists, and basic molecular scientists, mostly with close ties to the NCI. Many board members and their colleagues apply for and obtain funding from both the ACS and the NCI. Substantial NCI funds also go to ACS directors who sit on key NCI committees. Although the ACS asks board members to leave the room when the rest of the board discusses their funding proposals, this is just a token formality. In this private club, easy access to funding is one of the perks as the board routinely rubber-stamps approvals. A significant amount of ACS research funding goes to this extended membership. Frank conflicts of interest are evident in many ACS priorities. These include their advocating mammography and the National Breast Cancer Awareness campaign and supporting the pesticide and cancer drug industries. These conflicts even extend to the privatization of national cancer policy.

Public Relations

- 1998–2000: PR for the ACS was handled by Shandwick International whose major clients included RJ Reynolds Tobacco Holdings.
- 2000–2002: PR for the ACS was handled by the Edelman Public Relations, whose major clients included Brown & Williamson Tobacco Company, and the Altria Group, the parent company of Philip Morris, and Kraft.

Industry Funding

ACS has received contributions in excess of $100,000 from a wide range of "Excalibur donors." Some of these companies were responsible for environmental pollution with carcinogens while others manufactured and sold products containing toxic and carcinogenic ingredients. These include as follows:

- Petrochemical companies (DuPont, BP and Pennzoil)
- Industrial waste companies (BFI Waste Systems)
- Big Pharma (AstraZeneca, Bristol-Myers Squibb, GlaxoSmithKline, Merck & Company, and Novartis)
- Auto companies (Nissan and General Motors)
- Cosmetic companies (Christian Dior, Avon, Revlon, and Elizabeth Arden)
- Junk food companies (Wendy's International, McDonalds's, Unilever/Best Foods, and Coca-Cola)
- Biotech companies (Amgen and Genetech)

December 9, 2011

WHY WE ARE STILL LOSING THE WINNABLE WAR AGAINST CANCER

The Cancer Prevention Coalition is today calling for public scrutiny of the attitude taken by National Cancer Institute Director Harold Varmus toward the prevention of cancer. In a November 16, 2011 *Journal of the National Cancer Institute* article, "Why the US Has Gone Global in the Fight Against Cancer," Eric Rosenthal quotes Dr. Varmus as saying that he "wants us to look very carefully at what needs to be done in the areas of cancer research, cancer prevention – and broader issues of cancer control."

Varmus has a distinguished track record in basic research on cancer treatment, acknowledges Cancer Prevention Coalition Chairman Samuel S. Epstein, MD. However, as emphasized in a March 2010 Cancer Prevention Coalition press release, "this is paralleled by frank ignorance of well-documented and longstanding scientific evidence on cancer prevention."

Moreover, as long ago as 1998, Varmus claimed, "You can't do experiments to see what causes cancer – it's not an accessible problem, and not the sort of thing scientists can afford to do – everything you do can't be risky."

Contrary to Varmus, the International Agency for Research on Cancer (IARC) has published annual reports on carcinogens, largely based on carcinogenicity tests on rodents, since 1964. The National Toxicology Program (NTP) has also published, and continues to do so, systematic and comprehensive reviews on carcinogens, again largely based on carcinogenicity tests, since 1980. Dr. Epstein points out that "both the IARC and NTP reports detail decades-old unarguable scientific evidence on what causes cancer."

"The ignorance or indifference of Varmus to cancer prevention is reinforced by his unrecognized personal conflicts of interest," asserts Dr. Epstein. "In 1995, Varmus, then director of the National Institutes of Health, revoked the 'reasonable pricing clause,' which protected against exorbitant industry profiteering from the sale of drugs developed with taxpayer money."

Varmus also gave senior NCI staff free license to consult with the cancer drug industry, which Dr. Epstein terms, "a flagrant institutional conflict of interest." In this connection, the 2008 edition of the Charity Rating Guide & Watchdog Report listed Varmus with a compensation package of about $2.7 million. According to *The Chronicle of Philanthropy*, this is the highest compensation to directors in over 500 major non-profit organizations ever monitored.

As a past major recipient of NCI funds for basic genetic research, Varmus warned that "reasonable pricing" clauses, protecting against exorbitant industry profiteering from drugs developed with taxpayer dollars, were driving away private industry. So he struck these from agreements between industry and the NCI. "As a consequence," Dr. Epstein says, "Varmus has eliminated any price controls on cancer drugs made at the taxpayer expense."

"Illustratively," says Dr. Epstein, "using taxpayers' money, NCI paid for the research and development of Taxol, an anticancer drug manufactured by Bristol-Myers Squibb. Following completion of clinical trials, an extremely expensive process in itself, the public paid again for developing the drug's manufacturing process."

Once completed, the NCI gave Bristol-Myers Squibb the exclusive right to sell Taxol at an inflationary price, says Dr. Epstein, quoting the investigative journalist, Joel Bleifuss, who warned in a 1995 *In These Times* article, "Bristol-Myers Squibb sells Taxol to the public for $4.87 per milligram, which is more than 20 times what it costs to produce."

Taxol has been a blockbuster for Bristol-Myers, posting sales of over $3 billion since its approval in 1992, and accounting for about 40 percent of the company's sales.

"NCI Director Varmus still appears unconcerned that almost 700 carcinogens, to which the public is periodically or regularly exposed, have been identified and published in scientific journals by independent scientists," Dr. Epstein says. "He also seems unaware that the more cancer is prevented the less there is to treat."

Based on recent estimates by the National Institutes of Health, the total costs of cancer are about $219 billion each year. The annual costs to taxpayers of diagnosis and treatment amount to $89 billion; the annual costs of premature death are conservatively estimated at $112 billion; and the annual costs due to loss of productivity are conservatively estimated at $18 billion. "The human costs surely are of far greater magnitude. Much of these costs could be saved by cancer prevention," declares Dr. Epstein.

Examples of these avoidable cancers include:

- Breast cancer has increased by 21% due to a wide range of factors. These include: birth control pills; toxic hormonal ingredients in cosmetics and personal care products; diagnostic radiation; and routine premenopausal mammography, with a cumulative breast dose exposure of up to about five rads over ten years
- Malignant melanoma (mortality) of the skin in adults has increased by 185% due to the use of sunscreens in childhood that fail to block long wave ultraviolet light
- Thyroid cancer has increased by 168% due in large part to childhood dental and other radiation
- Non-Hodgkin's lymphoma has increased by 83% due mostly to phenoxy herbicides; and phenylenediamine hair dyes
- Testicular cancer has increased by 58% due to pesticides; hormonal ingredients in cosmetics and personal care products; and estrogen residues in meat;
- Childhood leukemia has increased by 42% due to ionizing radiation;

domestic pesticides; nitrite preservatives in meats, particularly hot dogs; and parental exposures to occupational carcinogens;

- Ovary cancer (mortality) for women over the age of 65 has increased by 39% in African American women and 10% in Caucasian women due to genital use of talc powder;

These concerns regarding Dr. Varmus have been recognized and endorsed by the following leading national experts on cancer prevention:

Rosalie Bertell, PhD
Regent, International Physicians for Humanitarian Medicine, Geneva, Switzerland
Past President of International Institute for Concern for Public Health

Ronnie Cummins
Executive Director, Organic Consumers Association

Janette D. Sherman, MD
New York Academy of Sciences, 2009

Quentin D. Young, MD
Chairman, Health and Medicine Policy Research Group
Past President of American Public Health Association

The American Cancer Society's Reckless, If Not Criminal, Track Record on Prevention of Breast and Other Cancers

1977 The ACS opposed regulations for hair coloring products that contained dyes known to cause breast and liver cancer in rodents.

The ACS also called for a Congressional moratorium on the FDA's proposed ban on saccharin and even advocated its use by nursing mothers and babies in "moderation," despite clear-cut evidence of its carcinogenicity in rodents. This reflects the consistent rejection by the ACS of the importance of animal evidence as predictive of human cancer risk.

1984 The ACS created the October National Breast Cancer Awareness Month, funded and promoted by Zeneca, an offshoot of the UK Imperial Chemical Industry, a major manufacturer of petrochemical products. The ACS leads women to believe that mammography is their best hope against breast cancer. A recent ACS advertisement promised that "early detection results in a cure nearly 100% of the time." Responding to questions from a journalist, an ACS communications director admitted: "The ad is based on a study. When you make an advertisement, you just say what you can to get women in the door. You exaggerate a point. Mammography today is a lucrative [and] highly competitive business." Even more seriously, the Awareness Month publications and advertisements studiously avoid any reference to the wealth of information on avoidable causes and prevention of breast cancer.

1989 Launched in 1989 by the Cosmetic, Toiletry, and Fragrance Association (CTFA) and the National Cosmetology Association, the Look Good . . . Feel Better Program was "dedicated to teaching women cancer patients beauty techniques to help restore their appearance and self-image during cancer treatment."

Just what could be more noble? Or so it might just seem. The October 2005 Look Good Program was supported by 22 CTFA-member cosmetic companies, including multibillion-dollar household name global giants. Each year, member companies "donate over one million individual cosmetic and personal care products, valued at $10 million, and raise more than $2 million." The Program was administered nationwide by the ACS, "which managed volunteer training, and served as the primary source of information to the public."

There is no doubt that the products donated by the cosmetic companies, such as eye and cheek colors, lipsticks, moisture lotions, pressed powders and other makeup, are restorative. However, there is also no doubt that the ACS and the companies involved were oblivious to or strangely silent on the dangers of the Look Good products, whose ingredients were readily absorbed through the skin.

A review of twelve Look Good products, marketed by six companies, revealed that ten contained toxic ingredients. These pose risks of cancer, and also hormonal (endocrine disruptive) effects.

Evidence for the cancer risks is based on standard tests in rodents, and on human (epidemiological) studies. Evidence for the hormonal risks is based on test-tube tests with breast cancer cells, or by stimulating premature sexual development in infant rodents. Unbelievably, the ACS explicitly warns women undergoing cancer chemotherapy—"Don't use hormonal creams."

Take, for example, Estee Lauder's LightSource Transforming Moisture Lotion, Chanel's Sheer Lipstick, and Merle Norman Eye Color. These products contain ingredients that are carcinogenic, contaminated with carcinogens, or precursors of carcinogens. The products also contain hormonal ingredients, known as parabens, one of which has been identified in breast cancer tissue, and incriminated as a probable cause of breast cancer.

The ACS's silence with regard to the risks of the Look Good products extends more widely to cosmetics and personal care products used by women, personal care products used by men, and baby lotions and shampoos. This silence is also consistent with the imbalanced objectives of the ACS annual and highly publicized "Breast Cancer Awareness Month." While dedicated to the early detection of breast cancer, this event is silent on a wide range of its avoidable causes, besides the escalating incidence of post-menopausal breast cancer, by nearly 40 percent, over the last three decades.

Of likely relevance to the ACS silence is its interlocking interests with the cosmetic, besides other industries. The major Look Good companies were among some 350 ACS "Excalibur Donors," each donating a minimum of $10,000 annually. Other donors include petrochemical, power plant, and hazardous waste industries, whose environmental pollutants have been incriminated as causes of breast and other cancers.

The ACS silence was also recklessly shared by the National Cancer Institute (NCI), which is required by the 1971 National Cancer Act to provide the public with information on avoidable causes of cancer. However, in spite of approximately $50 billion of taxpayers funding since 1971, the NCI has joined with the ACS in denying the public's right to know of avoidable causes of cancer from industrial chemicals, radiation, and common prescription drugs. Both the NCI and ACS are locked at the hip in policies fixated on damage control-screening, diagnosis, treatment, and treatment-related research, with indifference to cancer prevention due to avoidable exposures to chemical carcinogens in cosmetics, other consumer products, air, and water.

Equally asleep at the wheel remained the Food and Drug Administration in spite of its regulatory authority. The 1938 Federal Food, Drug and Cosmetic Act explicitly requires that "The label of cosmetic products shall bear a warning statement . . . to prevent a health hazard that may be associated with a product."

1992 The ACS issued a joint statement with the Chlorine Institute in support of the continued global use of organochlorine pesticides, despite clear evidence that some were known to cause breast cancer. In this statement, ACS vice president Clark Heath, MD, dismissed evidence of any risk as "preliminary and mostly based on weak and indirect association." Heath then went on to explain away the blame for increasing breast cancer rates as due to better detection: "Speculation that such exposures account for observed geographic differences in breast cancer occurrence should be received with caution; more likely, much of the recent rise in incidence in the United States . . . reflects increased utilization of mammography over the past decade."

In conjunction with the NCI, the ACS aggressively launched a "chemoprevention" program aimed at recruiting sixteen thousand healthy women at supposedly "high risk" of breast cancer into a five-year clinical trial with a highly profitable drug called tamoxifen. This drug is manufactured by one of the world's most powerful cancer drug industries, Zeneca, an offshoot of the Imperial Chemical Industries. The women were told that the drug was essentially harmless, and that it could reduce their risk of breast cancer. What the women were not told was that tamoxifen had already been shown to be a highly potent liver carcinogen in rodent tests, and also a well-known cause of uterine cancer.

1994 The ACS published a study designed to reassure women on the safety of dark permanent hair dyes and trivialize risks of fatal and nonfatal cancers, as documented in over six prior reports. However, the ACS study was based on a group of some 1,100 women with an initial age of fifty-six who were followed for seven years only. The ACS concluded that "women using permanent hair dyes are not generally at increased risk of fatal cancer." However, risks of cancer in women over sixty-three are up to twenty times higher for non-Hodgkin's lymphoma and multiple myeloma, thirty-four times for bladder cancer, and eight times for breast cancer. As designed, the ACS study would have missed the great majority of these cancers, and excluded dark hair dyes as important risks of avoidable cancers.

1998 In *Cancer Facts & Figures 1998*, the annual ACS publication designed to provide the public and medical profession with "Basic Facts" on cancer, there is little or no mention of prevention. Examples include: dusting the genital area with talc as a known cause of ovarian cancer; no mention of parental exposure to occupational carcinogens as a major cause of childhood cancer; prolonged use of oral contraceptives and hormone replacement therapy as major causes of breast cancer. For breast cancer, ACS stated: "Since women may not be able to alter their personal risk factors, the best opportunity for reducing mortality is through early detection." In other words, breast cancer is not preventable in spite of clear evidence that its incidence had escalated over recent decades, and in spite of an overwhelming amount of literature on its avoidable causes. In the section on "Nutrition and Diet," no mention is made of the heavy contamination of animal and dairy fats, and produce with a wide range of carcinogenic pesticide residues, and on the need to switch to safer organic foods.

The ACS allocated $330,000, under 0.1% of its $678 million revenues, to research on Environmental Carcinogenesis, while claiming allocations of $2.6 million, 0.4% of its revenues.

1999 The ACS denied any risks of cancer from drinking genetically-engineered (rBGH) milk. Its position has remained unchanged in spite of strong scientific evidence relating rBGH milk to major risks of breast, prostate, and colon cancers, as detailed in my 2006 book, *What's In Your Milk?* (Trafford Publishing, 2006).

Evidence for these risks is also summarized in my May 11, 2007, and January 12, 2010, Citizen Petitions to the Food and Drug Administration. These requested the FDA Commissioner "to label milk and other dairy products produced with the use of Posilac with a cancer risk warning." Both petitions were endorsed by leading national experts, and supported by over sixty scientific references. However, the FDA has still remained recklessly unresponsive.

CANCER	AUTHOR	INCREASED RISKS
BREAST	Bruning et al, 1995	7.3-fold
	Hankinson et al, 1998	7.3-fold
	Del Giudice et al, 1998	2.1-fold
PROSTATE	Signorello et al, 1999	5.1-fold
	Chan et al, 1998	4.3-fold
	Mantzoros et al, 1997	1.9-fold
	Wolk et al, 1995	1.4-fold
COLON	Pollak et al, 1999	5.0-fold
	Manousos et al, 1999	2.7-fold
	Ma et al, 1999	2.5-fold
	Giovanucci et al, 1999	2.2-fold

2002 In the *ACS Cancer Facts and Figures 2002*, the Community Cancer Control Section includes a "Look Good . . . Feel Better" program to teach women cancer patients beauty techniques to help restore their appearance and self-image during chemotherapy and radiation treatment." This program was partnered by the National Cosmetology Association and The Cosmetic, Toiletry and Fragrance Association Foundation, which failed to disclose the wide range of carcinogenic ingredients in toiletries and cosmetics. These trade organizations have also failed to disclose evidence of excess risks of breast and other cancers following long-term use of black or dark brown permanent and semi-permanent hair dyes. The ACS also failed to inform women of these avoidable risks.

The Environmental Cancer Risk Section of the *ACS Facts and Figures Report* also reassured that carcinogenic exposures from dietary pesticides, "toxic wastes in dump sites," ionizing radiation from "closely controlled" nuclear power plants, and non-ionizing radiation, are all "at such low levels that risks are negligible."

2008 The ACS indifference to cancer prevention has remained unchanged despite evidence on the escalating incidence of a wide range of cancers for over three decades, as documented by the National Toxicology Program and the International Agency for Cancer Research.

BREAST CARCINOGENS LISTED IN THE 2010 AMERICAN CANCER SOCIETY (ACS) REPORT AS "NEEDING MORE STUDY"

(Previously identified as carcinogens by the 2010 President's Cancer Panel [PCP] Report and by the 2004 National Toxicology Program [NTP] 11th Report on Carinogens)

Carcinogens	NTP (2004)*	PCP (2010)
Lead and Lead compounds	+	+
Diesel exhaust	+	++
Styrene-7,8-oxide & styrene	+	+
Propylene oxide	+	
Formaldehyde	+	++
Acetaldehyde	+	
Methylene chloride	+	+
Trichloroethylene	+	++
Tetrachloroethylene	+	+
Chloroform	+	++
Polychlorinated biphenyls	+	++

*NTP Rating
+ Reasonably anticipated

**PCP Rating
+ Suspected
++ Strong

2011 On February 18, the ACS stated that it has "no formal position regarding rBGH [in milk]" and that "the evidence for potential harm to humans is inconclusive." The ACS also claimed that "while there may be a link between IGF-1 levels in milk and cancer, the exact nature of this link remains unclear." This claim is also contrary to the unequivocal evidence of increased risks of breast, colon, and prostate cancers (see 1999 Track Record).

2012 The basic position of the ACS on the avoidable causes of cancer, other than predominantly lifestyle and smoking, remains unchanged. However, its 2012 Annual Report makes limited reference to risks of lung cancer from occupational exposure to certain heavy metals, organic chemicals, and radiation and risks of breast cancer from occupational exposures, as recognized by the International Agency for Research on Cancer.

AMERICAN CANCER SOCIETY, *CANCER FACTS & FIGURES 2012* *RISK FACTORS FOR BREAST CANCER*

Increasing Age
Obesity
Estrogen-Progestin (Hormonal therapy)
Physical Inactivity
1 or more alchoholic beverages daily
High-Dose Chest Radiation for Cancer Treatment
Early Menarche
Recent Use of Oral Contraceptives
Childlessness
Family History (BRCA 1 & 2 genes)
Smoking (Limited evidence)
Shift Work (Limited evidence)

INTERNATIONAL AGENCY FOR RESEARCH ON CANCER (IARC) LISTING OF CARCINOGENS INDUCING CANCERS, DECEMBER 2011

Carcinogen	Limited Evidence*	Sufficient Evidence**
Ethylene Oxide	Yes	
X-Radiation		Yes
Alcohol		Yes
Smoking	Yes	
Diethylstilbestrol		Yes
Estrogen-Progesterone Contraceptives		Yes
Estrogen-Progesterone Menopausal Therapy		Yes
Shift Work		Yes

*The data suggest a carcinogenic effect but are too limited for a definitive evalutaion
**A casual relationship has been established between the carcinogen and an increased incidence of breast cancer

National Academy of Sciences, December 2011 Report on Avoidable Causes of Breast Cancer

HORMONES
- Hormone therapy: androgens, estrogens, combined estrogen-progestin
- Oral contraceptives

BODY FATNESS AND ABDOMINAL FAT

ADULT WEIGHT GAIN

PHYSICAL INACTIVITY

DIETARY FACTORS
- Alcohol consumption
- Zeranol and zearalenone (estrogenic fungal toxin in beer)

TOBACCO SMOKE
- Active smoking
- Passive smoking

RADIATION
- Ionizing (including X-rays and gamma rays)
- Non-ionizing (extremely low frequency electromagnetic fields)

SHIFT WORK

METALS
- Aluminum
- Arsenic
- Cadmium
- Iron
- Lead
- Mercury

COSMETIC PRODUCTS AND INGREDIENTS
- Alkylphenols
- Bisphenol A (BPA)
- Nail products
- Hair dyes

- Parabens

INDUSTRIAL CHEMICALS
- Benzene
- 1,2-Butadiene
- PCBs
- Ethylene oxide
- Vinyl chloride
- Perfluorinated compounds (PFOA, PFOS)
- Phthlates
- Polybrominated diphenyl ethers (PBDEs; flame retardants)

PESTICIDES
- DDT/DDE
- Dieldrin and aldrin
- Atrazine and S-chloro triazine herbicides (atrazine)

POLYCYCLIC AROMATIC HYDROCARBONS

DIOXINS

Citizen Petitions to the Food and Drug Administration Authored by Dr. Epstein

MAY 12, 1995
CITIZEN PETITION SEEKING A MEDICAL ALERT FOR ALL WOMEN WITH SILICONE GEL AND POLYURETHANE BREAST IMPLANTS

MAY 11, 2007
CITIZEN PETITION SEEKING THE WITHDRAWAL OF THE NEW ANIMAL DRUG APPLICATION APPROVAL FOR POSILAC-RECOMBINANT BOVINE GROWTH HORMONE (RBGH) MILK (RESUBMITTED JANUARY 12, 2010)

May 12, 1995

CITIZEN PETITION SEEKING A MEDICAL ALERT FOR ALL WOMEN WITH SILICONE GEL AND POLYURETHANE BREAST IMPLANTS[76]

David A. Kessler, M.D.
Commissioner
Food and Drug Administration, Room 1-23
12420 Parklawn Drive
Rockville, MD 20857

The undersigned submits on behalf of the Cancer Prevention Coalition, Inc. (CPC), Samuel S. Epstein, M.D., Chair, and the Center for constitutional Rights, Michael Deutsch, Esq. Legal Director. This citizen petition is based on scientific publications dating back to 1960 which clearly demonstrate the carcinogenicity of silicone gel and polyurethane foam (PUF) breast implants. This evidence is further supported by internal Food and Drug Administration (FDA) memoranda.

The undersigned submits this petition under 21 USC. 321 (n), 361, 362, and 371 (a): and 21 CFR740.1, 740.2 of 21 CFR 10.30 of the Federal Food, Drug, and Cosmetic Act to request the Commissioner of Food and Drugs to issue a medical alert to all women who have had silicone gel breast implants with high priority to those with PUF implants, warning them of their risks of breast cancer and of the need for ongoing medical surveillance.

A. AGENCY ACTION REQUESTED

This petition requests that FDA take the following action:

(1) Immediately issue a medical alert to women who have received silicone gel and PUF breast implants, informing them of the risks of breast cancer.

(2) Pursuant to 21 CFR 10.30 (h) (2), a hearing at which time we can present our scientific evidence.

---

76 The FDA failed to respond to this petition.

B. STATEMENT OF GROUNDS

In April 1992, the FDA banned silicone gel breast implants except for use in controlled trials. This decision by the FDA was in response to serious questions raised concerning the health risks of implants. However, despite banning the general use of silicone implants, the agency failed to address the risks of cancer.

1. Carcinogenicity of Silicone Gel

An unpublished Dow Corning study discovered by the FDA in 1987, demonstrated that subcutaneous injection of silicone gel in rats induced highly malignant and metastatic fibrosarcomas.(1) Commenting on these findings, FDA Task Force scientists excluded the possibility that these could be solid state tumors;(2) it was further urged that "a medical alert be issued to warn the public of the possibility of malignancy development in humans following long-term implant of silicone breast prostheses." The carcinogenicity of silicone gel was subsequently confirmed following intra-peritoneal injection in mice.(3)

2. Carcinogenicity of Polyurethane Foam

In a series of publications from 1960 to 1964, Dr. Wilhelm Hueper (Chief of the Environmental Cancer Section at the National Cancer Institute) reported on the induction of carcinomas and/or sarcomas following intraperitoneal or subcutaneous injection of PUF in rats.(4,5,6,7) Apart from the induction of carcinomas, the possibility that the sarcomas could have been "solid state tumors" was definitively excluded. Furthermore, Hueper demonstrated the rapid in vivo degradation of PUF.

On the basis of these findings, Hueper warned:

- "Since polyurethane plastics have been used in cosmetic and orthopedic surgery during recent years, these observations are of distinct significance and practical importance,—(and) should caution against the indiscriminate use of polyurethane plastics in medical practice—."(4)
- "against indiscriminate parenteral use of polyurethane plastics—in medical practice."(5)
- "It is premature—to conclude from the present absence of carcinogenic

(human) responses—that the innocuousness of these materials—is established.—(as) any cancerous reaction—might require an induction period of some 30 years or more."(7)

On the basis of Hueper's studies, a senior FDA staff scientist concluded in 1991 that "PU[polyurethane] is acting as a straight-forward chemical carcinogen—and is not an appropriate material for use in breast implants."(8)

The carcinogenicity of PUF was subsequently confirmed by the induction of fibrosarcomas and carcinomas in rats following intraperitoneal and intrapulmonary administration, respectively.(9,10) The authors excluded the possibility that the sarcomas were "solid state tumors,"and emphasized that their findings were "consistent with a mechanism of biological degradation."(10)

3. Carcinogenicity of Contaminants and Degradation Products of Polyurethane Foam

2,4–Diaminotoluene (TDA) and 2,4–toluene diisocyanate (TDI) have been demonstrated to be carcinogenic contaminants and degradation products of PUF in both in vitro and in vivo studies.(11,12,13,14,15,15) Additionally, TDA has been identified in both the urine and breast milk of women with silicone gel breast implants.(17,18,19) It was accordingly concluded in 1994 that "TDA release from PU foam covers of—breast implants will undoubtedly produce delayed adverse health effects."(16)

The carcinogenicity of TDI in mice and rats was first reported in 1983. (20) Of particular interest was the induction of a statistically significant incidence of mammary fibroadenomas, besides malignant tumors in other sites in rats. On the basis of these data the International Agency for Research on Cancer (IARC) determined that there was "sufficient evidence" of TDI's carcinogenicity in mice and rats, including the induction of mammary tumors in female rats.(21) These conclusions were subsequently reiterated by the National Toxicological Program.(22) TDI is currently regulated by: the Environmental Protection Agency (EPA), under the Clean Air Act (CAA), Comprehensive Environmental, Response, Compensation and Liability Act (CERCLA), Resource Conservation and Recovery Act (RCRA), and Superfund Amendments and Reauthorization Act (SARA); the Occupational Safety and Health Administration (OSHA) under the Hazard

Communication Standard and as a Chemical Hazard in laboratories; and by the FDA as an indirect food additive.

There is substantial evidence on the carcinogenicity of TDA dating back to 1955. when it was found that subcutaneous injection induced local sarcomas in rats.(23) Invasive and metastatic liver cancer was subsequently induced in rats fed with TDA.(24) It is worthy of note that on the basis of these data, the cosmetic industry voluntarily eliminated the use of TDA in hair dyes in 1971. A statistically significant incidence of benign and malignant mammary tumors was induced in rats fed with TDA;(25) these tumors developed after only one month feeding. A statistically significant incidence of liver cancer and vascular tumors was induced in mice, and benign and malignant breast tumors, besides tumors in other sites, were induced in rats following feeding of TDA.(26) On the basis of these data, IARC concluded that there was "sufficient evidence" of the carcinogenicity of TDA in mice and rats.(27) These conclusions were reiterated by the National Toxicology Program, which further warned that "the presence of TDA, even as a trace contaminant, may be a cause of cancer."(28)

TDA is currently regulated by EPA as a priority hazardous substance under SARA; OSHA under the Hazard Communication Standard as a Chemical Hazard in laboratories; and by the FDA which requires warning labels on coal tar hair dyes containing TDA under the Federal Food, Drug, and Cosmetic Act.

An unpublished Congressionally-mandated NCI report emphasized that concerns on "a carcinogenic hazard were recently heightened by reports that the polyurethane foam coating that envelopes the silica gel—may dissolve and produce the chemical 2,4 diaminotoluene (TDA)—linked to increased rates of breast and hepatocellular carcinomas in rats and mice and possibly also sarcomas and lymphomas in mice."(29)

4. Carcinogenicity of Ethylene Oxide

Ethylene oxide (ETO) has been routinely used to sterilize breast implants. A July 11, 1988 FDA audit of Cooper Surgical revealed a wide range of deficiencies in control procedures, including the absence of formalized procedures for methods for sterilization and aeration, and for failure to test for residues. These concerns are of particular significance as

ETO residues are known to persist on medical products, including plastics, even after seven days aeration.(30,31) ETO is a well-recognized carcinogen inducing breast cancer, malignant lymphomas and other cancers in mice, and leukemia, brain tumors and other cancers in rats following inhalation, and fibrosarcomas in mice following subcutaneous injection.(32)

5. Epidemiological studies on Women with Silicone Breast Implants

Based on a cohort of 11,676 women in Alberta receiving silicone gel or saline implants from 1973 to 1986, with a mean follow-up of only 10.2 years, a deficit of breast cancer was reported. PU implants were not used in Alberta during the study period.(33) In a subsequent study with a median follow-up of only 10.6 years, deficits of breast cancer in implanted women and of all other malignancies combines were reported. However, based on small numbers, an increased incidence of lung, vulva, and invasive cervical carcinomas, were reported.(34)

However, as emphasized by an NCI report, these studies are seriously flawed and clearly not exculpatory.(35) Furthermore, NCI urged longitudinal studies on women with various types of implants. NCI stated: "This call for further study reflects the paucity of available data on long-term effects of augmentation mammaplasty. Most studies evaluating breast cancer risk have lacked systematic case ascertainment and estimates of expected risk. In the two large-scale epidemiologic studies, only scant information on possible disease covariates was available, limiting the ability to evaluate observed relationships. In addition, the devices evaluated were for the most part markedly different in design and material from those currently in use. Thus, further follow-up of a large cohort of women is needed, with particular attention given to effects of specific types of implants.(35) Senior FDA scientists have also confirmed that sufficient time has not elapsed to record epidemiologically significant increases in human malignancies involving silicone gel implants.(2)

C. CLAIM FOR CATEGORICAL EXCLUSION

A claim for categorical exclusion is asserted pursuant to 21 CFR 25.24 (a) (11).

D. CERTIFICATION

The undersigned certifies, that, to the best knowledge and belief of the undersigned, this petition includes all information and views on which the petition relies, and that it includes representatives data and information known to the petitioner which are unfavorable to the petition.

This petition is submitted by:

Samuel S. Epstein, M.D.

Chairman, Cancer Prevention Coalition

Professor Occupational and Environmental Medicine

University of Illinois School of Public Health, Chicago

Michael Deutsch, Esq.

Legal Director, Center for Constitutional Rights, New York

REFERENCES

1. FED. Reg. 55:20568–20577, 5/17/90
2. FDA staff scientists Drs. Lorentzen, Luu, Sheridan & Stratmeyer. Internal agency memoranda, August and September, 1988.
3. Potter, Journal of the National Cancer Institute, 86:1058–1065, 1994.
4. Hueper, Journal of the American Medical Association, 173:860, 1960.
5. Hueper, American Journal of Clinical Pathology, 34:334–337, 1960.
6. Hueper, Pathol. Microbiol. 24:77–106, 1961.
7. Hueper, Journal of the National Cancer Institute, 33:1005–1027, 1964.
8. Mishra, April 1991, Memo to the Director, FDA Office of Device Evaluation.
9. Autian et al, Cancer Res. 35:1591–1596, 1975.
10. Autian et al, Cancer Res. 36:3973–3977, 1976.
11. Guthrie & McKinney, Anl. Chem. 49:1676–1680, 1977.
12. Batich et al. J. Biomed. Mater. Res. 23:311–319, 1989.
13. Guidoin et al, Ann. Plastic Surg. 28:342–353, 1992.
14. Amin et al (Bristol Myers), J. Biomed. Mater. Res. 27:655–666, 1993.
15. Benoit, J. Biomed.. Mater. Res. 27:1341–1348, 1993.
16. Luu et al. J. Appl. biomater. 5:1–7, 1994.
17. Chan et al, Clin. Chem. 37/12:756–758, 1991.
18. Chan et al, Clin. Chem. 37/2:2143–2145, 1991.
19. Aegis Analytical Laboratories, Press Release: 2,4-TDA Analysis with Regards to PUF Breast Implants, 6/4/91.
20. National Toxicology Program, NTP Carcinogenesis Tech. Report No. 82–2, 1983.
21. International Agency for Research on Cancer, 39:287–323, 1986.
22. National Toxicology Program, Seventh Annual Report on Carcinogens, Summary, 383–387, 1994.
23. Umeda, Gann 46:597–603, 1955.

24. Ito et al, Cancer Res. 29:1137–1145, 1969.
25. DuPont, Phenylenediamines, Unpublished Report to the Office of Toxic Substances, EPA, 1974.
26. Weisburger et al, J. Environ. Pathol. Toxicol. 2:325–326, 1978.
27. International Agency for Research on Cancer, 19:303–340, 1979.
28. National Toxicology Program, Seventh Annual Report on Carcinogens, Summary, 143–146, 1994.
29. Brinton, National Cancer Institute, Protocol for a Follow-Up Study of Women with Augmentation Mammaplasty, Report to Congress, 11/93.
30. International Agency for Research on Cancer, 19/36:189–226, 1985.
31. Agency of Toxic Substances and Disease Registry, (DHHS), A Toxicological Profile for Ethylene Oxide, 63–64, 1990.
32. National Toxicology Program, Seventh Annual Report on Carcinogens, Summary, 205–210, 1994.
33. Berkel et al. New England Journal of medicine, 326:1649–1653, 1992.
34. Deapen & Brody, Plastic Reconstr. Surg. 89:660–665, 1992.
35. Brinton, National Cancer Institute, Protocol for a Follow-up Study of Women with Augmentation Mammaplasty, Report to Congress, 11/93.

FDA RESPONSE (FEBRUARY 13, 1997)

Petition denied in view of the fact that "There is no evidence that has clearly linked these materials with cancer in humans."

May 11, 2007

CITIZEN PETITION SEEKING THE WITHDRAWAL OF THE NEW ANIMAL DRUG APPLICATION APPROVAL FOR POSILAC®-RECOMBINANT BOVINE GROWTH HORMONE (RBGH) MILK[77]

Mike Leavitt
Secretary of Health and Human Services
US Department of Health and Human Services

Andrew C. von Eschenbach, M.D.
Commissioner of Food and Drugs
Dockets Management Branch
Food and Drug Administration, Room 1061
5630 Fishers Lane
Rockville, MD 20852

---

77. The FDA failed to respond to this Petition, which was resubmitted on January 12, 2010, to which the FDA again failed to respond.

The undersigned submits this petition on behalf of the Cancer Prevention Coalition, Samuel S. Epstein, M.D., Chair; the Organic Consumers Association, Ronnie Cummins, Executive Director; Family Farm Defenders, John Kinsman, President; Arpad Pusztai, PhD, FRSE; and Institute for Responsible Technology, Jeffrey M. Smith, Executive Director.

This petition is based on scientific evidence of increased risks of cancer, particularly breast, colon, and prostate, from the consumption of milk from cows injected with Posilac®, the genetically modified recombinant bovine growth hormone (also known as rBGH, sometribove, recombinant bovine somatotropin, or rBST). Posilac® is the trademark for Monsanto's rBGH product, registered with the US Patent and Trademark Office, and is approved for marketing by the Food and Drug Administration (FDA). This petition is also based on abnormalities in the composition of rBGH milk, resulting from the recognized veterinary toxicity of rBGH, particularly increased levels of IGF-1.

The undersigned submit this petition under section 512(e)(1) of the Federal Food, Drug, and Cosmetic Act (21 USC. 360b(e)(1)(A)), to request the Secretary to immediately suspend approval of Posilac® based on imminent hazard; and under section 21 USC. 321 (n), 361, 362, and 371 (a), 21 CFR 740.1, 740.2 of 21 CFR 10.30 of the Federal Food, Drug, and Cosmetic Act to request the Commissioner of the Food and Drug Administration to label milk and other dairy products produced with the use of Posilac® with a cancer risk warning.

A. AGENCY ACTION REQUESTED

This petition requests the Secretary and the Commissioner to take the following action:

Suspend approval of Posilac®, and/or require milk and other dairy products produced with the use of Posilac® to be labeled with warnings such as, "Produced with the use of Posilac®, and contains elevated levels of IGF-1, a major risk factor for breast, prostate, and colon cancers."

B. STATEMENT OF GROUNDS

1. The Veterinary Toxicity of Posilac®

Evidence of these toxic effects was first detailed in confidential Monsanto reports, based on records of secret nationwide rBGH veterinary trials, submitted to the FDA prior to October 1989 when they were leaked to one of the petitioners, Dr. Epstein. He then made these reports available to Congressman John Conyers, Chairman of the House Committee on Government Operations. On May 8, 1990, Congressman Conyers issued the following statement. "I find it reprehensible that Monsanto and the FDA have chosen to suppress and manipulate animal health test data" (1). Details of these toxic effects were subsequently admitted by Monsanto and the FDA, and disclosed on the drug's veterinary label (Posilac®) in November, 1993. These include injection site lesions, a wide range of other toxic effects, and an increased incidence of mastitis, requiring the use of medication and antibiotics, and resulting in their contamination of milk.

2. Abnormalities in rBGH Milk

In a Monsanto Executive Summary, Posilac, January 1994, it was claimed that "natural milk is indistinguishable" from rBGH milk and that "There is no legal basis requiring its labeling." However, there are a wide range of well-documented abnormalities in rBGH milk, apart from increased IGF-1 levels (2–11). These include: reduction in casein; reduction in short-chain fatty acid and increase in long-chain fatty acid levels; increase in levels of the thyroid hormone triiodothyronine enzyme; contamination with unapproved drugs from treating mastitis; and frequency of pus cells due to mastitis.

3. Increased Levels of IGF-1 in rBGH Milk

A wide range of publications have documented excess levels of IGF-1 in rBGH milk (10–22), with increases ranging from four- to 20-fold. Based on six unpublished industry studies, FDA admitted that IGF-1 levels in rBGH milk were consistently and statistically increased, and that these were further increased by pasteurization (16); these increases were also admitted by others (17, 18). Included among these is one by Lilly Industries, in its application for marketing authorization to the European Community Committee for Veterinary Products, admitting that rBGH milk may contain more than 10-fold increase in IGF-1 levels (20). It should also be noted that pasteurization increases IGF-1 levels by a further 70% (16), presumably by disrupting protein binding, and since standard analytic techniques for IGF-1 in rBGH milk may underestimate its levels by up to 40-fold (9, 15).

4. IGF-1 Is Readily Absorbed from the Intestine into the Blood

Contrary to Section 2 of FDA's 6/8/2000 Docket No. 98P-1194 response to the December 5, 1998 Citizen Petition of the Center for Food Safety, IGF-1 is a peptide and not a protein, and as such is readily absorbed into the blood. Even more compelling is evidence of marked growth promoting effects following short-term feeding tests in rats (16, 22). FDA's Section 2 thus reflects a misunderstanding relating to "the possibility of IGF-1 surviving digestion."

5. Increased IGF-1 Levels Increase Risks of Breast, Colon and Prostate Cancers

Thus, increased levels of IGF-1 have been shown to increase risks of breast cancer by up to seven-fold in 19 publications (23–41), risks of colon cancer in 10 publications (42–51), and prostate cancer in 7 publications (52–57).

6. Increased IGF-1 Levels Inhibit Apoptosis

Of generally unrecognized, critical importance is the fact that increased IGF-1 levels block natural defense mechanisms against the growth and development of early submicroscopic cancers, known as apoptosis or programmed self destruction (53, 58, 59).

7. Bovine Growth Hormone Increases Twinning Rates

As increased rate of twinning in cows injected with rBGH was admitted by Monsanto on its November 1993 Posilac label. rBGH increases ovulation and embryo survival, and increases the incidence of fraternal twins (60). "Because multiple gestations are more prone to complications such as premature delivery, congenital defects and pregnancy-induced hypertension in the mother than singleton pregnancies, the findings of this study suggest that women contemplating pregnancy might consider substituting meat and dairy products with other protein sources, especially in countries that allow growth hormone administration to cattle" (61).

8. The International Ban on the Use and Imports of rBGH Dairy Products

Based on the veterinary and public health concerns detailed in this Petition, the use and import of rBGH dairy products has been banned by Canada, 29 European nations, Norway, Switzerland, Japan, New Zealand, and Australia.

It should further be noted that on June 30, 1999, the Codex Alimentarius Commission, the United Nations Food Safety Agency representing 101 nations worldwide, ruled unanimously not to endorse or set a safety standard for rBGH milk.

9. The FDA Policy on Labeling rBGH Milk

The FDA has misled dairy producers and consumers with regard to its requirement for labeling of rBGH milk, to the effect that "No significant difference has been shown between milk derived from rBST-treated and non-rBST treated cows." This, however, is misleading in extreme as the "FDA has determined it lacks the basis for requiring such labeling in its statute." This was admitted in a 7/27/94 letter by Jerold R. Mande, Executive Director to the FDA Commissioner, to Harold Rudnick, State of New York Department of Agriculture and Markets.

C. CLAIM FOR CATEGORICAL EXCLUSION

A claim for categorical exclusion is asserted pursuant to 21 CFR 25.24 (a)11.

D. CERTIFICATION

The undersigned certify, that, to their best knowledge and belief, this petition includes all information and views on which the petition relies, and also that it includes representative data and information known to the petitioner which are unfavorable to the petition.

This petition is submitted by:

Samuel S. Epstein, M.D.
Chairman, Cancer Prevention Coalition
Professor emeritus Occupational and Environmental Medicine
University of Illinois at Chicago

Ronnie Cummins
Executive Director
Organic Consumers Association

John Kinsman
President
Family Farm Defenders

Arpad Pusztai, Ph.D., FRSE

Jeffrey Smith
Executive Director
Institute for Responsible Technology

REFERENCES

1. Conyers, John. Letter to Richard R. Kusserow, Inspector General, Department of Health and Human Services. May 9, 1990.
2. Kennelly J & DeBoer G. Bovine somatotropin. In Proceedings of the Alberta Dairy Seminar. Banff, Alberta, March 9–11, 1998.
3. Baer RJ, et al. Composition and flavor of milk produced by cows injected with recombinant bovine somatotropin. *Journal of Dairy Science* 72:1424–1434, 1989.
4. Capuco AV et al. Somatotropin increases thyroxine-5'-monodeiodinase activity in lactating mammary tissue of the cow. *Journal of Endocrinology* 121(2):205–211, 1989.
5. Epstein SS. Potential public health hazards of biosynthetic milk hormones. *International Journal of Health Services* 20:73–84, 1990.
6. Kronfeld DS. Safety of bovine growth hormone. Science 251:256–257, 1991.
7. US General Accounting Office. rBGH. FDA Approval Should Be Withheld Until the Mastitis Issues is Resolved. 1992.
8. Mepham TB. Public health implications of bovine somatotropin use in dairying: discussion paper. *Journal of the Royal Society of Medicine* 85:736–739, 1992.
9. Millstone E, et al. Plagiarism or protecting public health? Nature 371:647–648, 1994.
10. US General Accounting Office. Recombinant bovine growth hormone. FDA approval should be withheld until the mastitis issue is resolved. 1992.
11. Davis SR, et al. Effects of injecting growth hormone of thyroxine on milk production and blood plasma concentrations of insulin-like growth factors I and II in dairy cows. *Journal of Endocrinology* 114:17–24, 1987.
12. Prosser CG, et al. Changes in concentrations of IGF-1 in milk during BGH treatment in the goat. *Journal of Endocrinology* 112 (March Supplement): Abstract 65, 1987.
13. McBride BW, et al. The influence of bovine growth hormone (somatotropin) on animals and their products. *Research and Development in Agriculture* 5:1–21, 1988.
14. Francis GL, et al. Insulin-like growth factors 1 and 2 in bovine colostrum. Sequences and

biological activities compared with those of a potent truncated dorm. *Biochem J.* 251:95–103, 1988.

15. Prosser CG, et al, Increased secretion of insulin-like growth factor-1 into milk of cows treated with recombinantly derived bovine growth hormones. *Journal of Dairy Research* 56:17–26, 1989.

16. Juskevich JC & Guyer CG. Bovine growth hormone food safety evaluation. *Science* 249:875–884, 1990.

17. National Institutes of Health. Technology Assessment Conference Statement on Bovine Somatotropin. *Journal of the American Medical Association* 265:1423–1425, 1991.

18. Joint FAO/WHO Expert Committee on Food Additives (JECFA). Fortieth Report, Geneva. June 9–18, 1992. Cited six unpublished industry studies confirming increased IGF-1levels in rBGH milk. These included one by Monsanto (Schams et al, 1988) reporting a four-fold increases, and another (Miller et al, 1989) reporting a further 50% increase following pasteurization.

19. Epstein SS. BST and cancer. *New Scientist U.K.*, October 29, 1994.

20. Mepham TB, et al. Safety of milk from cows treated with bovine somatotropin. *The Lancet* 2:197, 1994.

21. Mepham TB & Schofield, PN. *International Dairy Federation Nutrition Week*, Paris, June 1995.

22. Epstein SS. Unlabeled milk from cows treated with biosynthetic growth hormones: a case of regulatory abdication. *International Journal of Health Services* 261:173–185, 1996.

23. Furlanetto RW & DiCarlo JN. Somatotropin-C receptors and growth effects in human breast cells maintained in long-term tissue culture. *Cancer Research* 44:2122–2128, 1984.

24. Glimm DR, et al. Effect of bovine somatotropin in the distribution of immunoreactive insulin-like growth factor-1 in lactating bovine mammary tissue. *Journal of Dairy Science* 71:2923–2935, 1988.

25. Reynolds RK, et al. Regulation of epidermal growth factor and insulin-like growth factors I receptors by estradiol and progesterone in normal and neoplastic endometrial cells cultures. *Gynecology Oncology* 38:396–406, 1990.

26. Lippman A. Growth factors, receptors and breast cancer. *National Institutes of Health Research* 3:59–62, 1991.

27. Rosen N, et al. Insulin-like growth factors in human breast cancer. *Breast Cancer Research Treatment* 18(Suppl):555–562, 1991.

28. Harris JR, et al. Breast Cancer. *New England Journal of Medicine* 7:473–480, 1992.

29. Pollak MN, et al. Tamoxifen reduced insulin-like growth factor-1 (IGF-1). *Breast Cancer Research Treatment* 22:91–100, 1992.

30. Lippman ME. The development of biological therapies for breast cancer. *Science* 259:631–632, 1993.

31. Pappa V, et al. Insulin-like growth factor-1 receptors are over expressed and predict a low risk in human breast cancer. *Cancer Research* 53:3736–3740, 1993.

32. Bruning PF, et al. Insulin-like growth factor-binding protein 3 is decreased in early-stage operable pre-menopausal breast cancer. *International Journal of Cancer* 62(3):266–270, July 1995.

33. Epstein SS. Unlabeled milk from cows treated with biosynthetic growth hormones: a case of regulatory abdication. *International Journal of Health Services* 261:173–185, 1996.

34. LeRoith D. Insulin-like growth factors and cancer. *Annals of Internal Medicine* 122(1):54–59, January 1995.

35. Bohlke K, et al. Insulin-like growth factor-1 in relation to premenopausal ductal carcinoma in situ of the breast. *Epidemiology* 9(5):570–573, 1998.

36. Del Giudice ME, et al. Insulin and related factors in premenopausal breast cancer risk. *Breast Cancer Research and Treatment* 47(2):111–120, 1998.

37. Hankinson SE, et al. Circulating concentrations of insulin-like growth factor-1 and risk of breast cancer. *The Lancet* 351:1393–1396, 1998.

38. Agurs-Collins T, et al. Insulin-like growth factor-1 and breast cancer risk in post-menopausal American women. Proceedings of the American Association of Cancer Research 40:152, 1999.

39. Toniolo P, et al. Serum insulin-like growth factor-1 and breast cancer. *International Journal of Cancer* 88(5):828–832, 2000.

40. Yu H & Rohan T. role of the insulin-like growth factor family in cancer development and progression. *Journal of the National Cancer Institute* 92:1472–1484, 2000.

41. Epstein SS. Re Role of the insulin-like growth factors in cancer development and progression. *Journal of the National Cancer Institute* 93(3):238, 2001.

42. Pines A, et al. Gastrointestinal tumors in acromegalic patients. *Am J Gastroenterology* 80:266–269, 1985.

43. Orme SM, et al. Cancer incidence and mortality in acromegaly: a retrospective cohort study. *Journal of Endocrinology Supplement* Number OC22, June 1996.

44. Epstein SS. Unlabeled milk from cows treated with biosynthetic growth hormones: a case of regulatory abdication. *International Journal of Health Services* 261:173–185, 1996.

45. Manousos O, et al. IGF-1 and IGF-II in relation to colorectal cancer. *International Journal of Cancer* 83:15–17, 1999.

46. Ma J, et al. Prospective study of colorectal cancer risk in men and plasma levels of insulin-like growth factor-1 and IGF-1 binding protein-3. *Journal of the National Cancer Institute* 91:620–625, 1999.

47. Giovannucci E, et al. Plasma insulin-like growth factor-I and binding protein-3 and risk of colorectal cancer and adenoma in women. Proceedings of the American Association of Cancer Research 40:211, 1999.

48. Renehan AG, et al. Circulating insulin-like growth factor II and colorectal adenomas. *Journal of Clinical Endocrinology & Metabolism* 85(9):3402–3408, 2000.

49. Pollak M, et al. Relationship of colorectal cancer risk to serum insulin-like growth factor I and insulin-like growth factor binding protein 3 levels [abstract]. Late breaking session. Philadelphia (PA): 90th annual meeting of the American Association for Cancer Research; April 10–14, 1999.

50. Juul A, et al. The ratio between serum levels of IGF-1 and the IGF binding protein decreases with age in healthy patients and is increased in acromegalic patients. *Clinical Endocrinology* 41:85–93, 1994.

51. Tremble JM & McGregor AM. In Treating Acromegaly, editor Wass p. 5–12. *Journal of Endocrinology Ltd.*, Bristol, England, 1994.

52. Mantzoros CS, et al. Insulin-like growth factor i in relation to prostate cancer and benign prostatic hyperplasia. *British Journal of Cancer* 76:1115–1118, 1997.

53. Chan JM, et al. Plasma insulin-like growth factor-I and prostate cancer risk: a prospective study. *Science* 279:563–566, 1998.

54. Wolk A, et al. Insulin-like growth factor 1 and prostate cancer risk: a population-based, case-control study. *Journal of the National Cancer Institute* 90:911–915, 1998.

55. Signorello LB, et al. Insulin-like growth factor-binding protein-1 and prostate cancer. *Journal of the National Cancer Institute* 91:1965–1967, 1999.

56. Stattin P, et al. Plasma insulin-like growth factor-binding proteins, and prostate cancer risk: a prospective study. *Journal of the National Cancer Institute* 92:1910–1917, 2000.

57. Harman SM, et al. Serum levels of insulin-like growth factor I (IGF-1), IGF-II, IGF-binding protein-3, and prostate-specific antigen as predictors of clinical prostate cancer. *Journal of Clinical Endocrinology & Metabolism* 85(11):4258–4265, 2000.

58. Resnicoff M, et al. The insulin-like growth factor I receptor protects tumor cells from apoptosis in vivo. *Cancer Research* 55(11):2463–2469, June 1, 1995.

59. Perks CM, et al. Differential IGF-independent effects of insulin-like growth factor binding proteins (1-6) on apoptosis of breast epithelial cells. *J Cell Biochem* 75:652–664, 1999.

60.   Steinman G. Mechanisms of twinning VII. Effect of diet and heredity on the human twinning rate. *Journal of Reproductive Medicine* 51(5):405–410, May 2006.

61.   "Study by LIJ Obstetrician Finds That A Woman's Chances of Having Twins Can Be Modified by Diet." Press release, North Shore Long Island Jewish Health System, June 7, 2006, http://www.northshorelij.com

Acknowledgments

The *International Journal of Health Services* (*IJHS*) over is unarguably a leading public health journal. Apart from rigorous scientific standards, its predominant emphasis is on the critical relation between public health science, public health policy, and human rights.

It is my privilege and pleasure to have published extensively in the *IJHS* over past decades. This book, *Stop Breast Cancer Before It Starts*, is based in part on my previous IJHS publications.

Apart from press releases and newspaper articles, this book is based in part on my 2005 *IJHS* book, *Cancer Gate: How To Win the Losing War Against Cancer.*

Warm commendations are due to Congressman John Conyers, Jr., former Chairman of the House Judiciary Committee, for his longstanding public health policy initiatives, and my 1979 invitation to draft legislation on "white-collar crime" in relation to industry malpractice. This crime knowingly exposes millions of unsuspecting citizens to avoidable risks of cancer from a wide range of industrial chemicals, ingredients in consumer products, and drugs. In 1981, Congressman Conyers warned that, "Monsanto and the Food and Drug Administration (FDA) have chosen to suppress and manipulate animal health test data in efforts to approve commercial use of rBGH, genetically engineered milk." He also endorsed my 2006 *What's In Your Milk?* book, which warned of the risks of breast, besides other cancers, from genetically engineered (rBGH) milk, dangers still criminally ignored by the Food and Drug Administration.

Thanks are also due to Dr. Quentin D. Young, former President of the American Public Health Association and Chairman of the Health and Medicine Policy Research Group, for his longstanding emphasis on the critical, but infrequently exercised, role of physicians in public health policy, and cancer prevention.

It is a pleasure to acknowledge the over one hundred scientific experts in cancer prevention and public health, and the over two hundred representatives of consumer and citizen activist groups, who endorsed the Cancer Prevention Coalition (CPC) February 2003 report, "Stop Cancer Before It Starts Campaign: How to Win the Losing War Against Cancer." It is also a pleasure to acknowledge the leading scientific experts who endorsed my 2007 FDA Citizen Petition on hormonal milk, and my 1995 and 2010 Petitions on the risks of breast cancer from nitrite-preservatives and hormonal meat.

I would also like to thank my research assistant, Alessandra Elder, for her strong interest and creative support.

About the Author

Samuel S. Epstein, MD is professor emeritus of Environmental and Occupational Medicine at the University of Illinois School of Public Health, and Chairman of the Cancer Prevention Coalition. He has published some 270 peer reviewed articles, and authored twenty books.

Dr. Epstein is an internationally recognized authority on avoidable causes of cancer, particularly unknowing exposures to industrial carcinogens in air, water, the workplace, and consumer products—food, cosmetics and toiletries, and household products including pesticides—besides carcinogenic prescription drugs.

Dr. Epstein's past public policy activities include: consultant to the US Senate Committee on Public Works; drafting Congressional legislation; frequently invited Congressional testimony; membership of key federal committees including EPA's Health Effects Advisory Committee, and the Department of Labor's Advisory Committee on the Regulation of Occupational Carcinogens; and key expert on banning of hazardous products and pesticides including DDT, Aldrin and Chlordane. He is the leading international expert on cancer risks of petrochemicals and of consumer products including: rBGH milk; meat from cattle implanted with sex hormones in feedlots, on which he has testified for the E.C. at January 1997 WTO hearings; and irradiated food. In 1998, he presented "Legislative Proposals for Reversing the Cancer Epidemic" to the Swedish Parliament, and in 1999 to the UK All Parliamentary Cancer Group. He has also submitted eight Citizen Petitions to the US Food and Drug Administration on the undisclosed dangers of carcinogens and carcinogenic products. These include: talc, lindane, nitrite-preserved foods, silicone gel and polyurethane implants, cosmetics containing DEA, genetically-engineered milk (rBGH), and hormonal beef.

He is also the leading critic of the cancer establishment, the National Cancer Institute (NCI) and American Cancer Society (ACS), for fixation on damage control—screening, diagnosis and treatment, and genetic research—with indifference for cancer prevention, which for the ACS extends to hostility. This mindset is compounded by ACS conflicts of interest with the cancer drug industry, and also with the petrochemical and other industries. The ACS thus qualifies for Ralph Nader's 1975 adage, "Jail for crime in the streets, [but] bail for crime in the suites."

Dr. Epstein past professional society involvement includes: founder of the Environmental Mutagen Society; President of the Society for Occupational and Environmental Health; President of the Rachel Carson Council; and advisor to environmental, citizen activist and organized labor groups.

His honors include: the 1969 Society of Toxicology Achievement Award; the 1977 National Wildlife Federation Conservancy Award; the 1989 Environmental Justice Award; the 1998 Right Livelihood Award ("Alternative Nobel Prize") for international contributions to cancer prevention; the 1999 Bioneers Award; the 2000 Project Censored Award ("Alternative Pulitzer Prize" for investigative journalism) for an article critiquing the American Cancer Society and National Cancer Institute; the 2005 Albert Schweitzer Golden Grand Medal for Humanitarianism from the Polish Academy of Medicine; and the 2007 Dragonfly Award from Beyond Pesticides.

Dr. Epstein has extensive media experience with: numerous regional and national radio programs, including NPR; major TV programs, including *60 Minutes*, *Face the Nation*, *Meet the Press*, *McNeil/Lehrer*, *Donohue*, *Good Morning America*, and the *Today Show*; Canadian, European, Australian and Japanese TV. He has also published about ten articles in leading national newspapers, and about 150 press releases, and forty *Huffington Post* blogs over the last two decades.